AF601878

Question Bank of
Biochemistry

The Authors

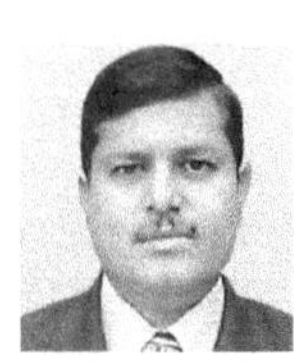

Dr. Nawaz Ahmad Khan obtained his M.Sc. (Ag) Biochemistry from N.D.U.A.& T, Kumarganj Faizabad. He did his Ph.D (Biochemistry) from Gujarat Agril. University, Junagarh in year 2000. His area of interest is Biotic stress in plants. He honored 'Young Scientist Award' 2013 by Alumni Association of N.D.U.A.T. Kumarganj.He got several Prizes and Honour in various National as well as International Conference. Currently he is working as Assistant Professor, Department of Biotechnology, N.D.U.A.&T. Kumarganj, Faizabad, U.P.

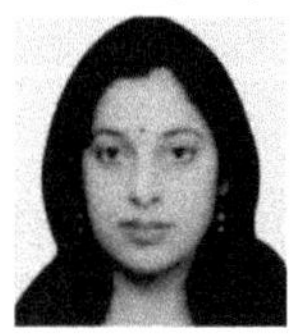

Dr. Pramila Pandey obtained her Ph.D. (Botany) from Dr. RML Awadh University, Faizabad. She qualified NET. She has P.G. Diploma in Bioinformatics. Presently Dr. Pandey is working as Programme Assistant in the Department of Biotechnology at N.D. University of Agriculture and Technology, Kumarganj, Faizabad.

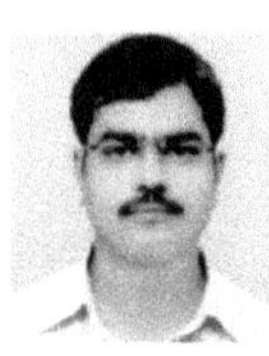

Dr. Md. Shamim did his M.Sc. Biotechnology and Ph.D. from NDUAT Faizabad. He had published various national and international papers in reputed journals as well as reviewed various research papers. Presently he is working as an Assistant Professor cum Junior Scientist (Biotechnology) in Bihar Agricultural University, Sabour, Bhagalpur.

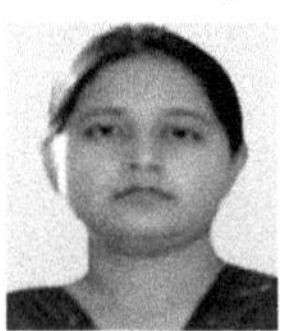

Deepti Srivastava completed her M.Sc. (Ag.) Biotechnology from NDUAT, Faizabad. She got DBT fellowship during PG programme also qualified NET. She did Ph.d (Ag.)Biotechnology from NDUAT, Faizabad. Presently she is engaged in research work on Gene pyramiding in Rice NDUAT, Faizabad.

Question Bank of
Biochemistry

for Ready Reference to the Students, Teachers and Researchers for NET, SET, Ph.D., JRF, SRF, Civil Service Examinations (State and Central) and other related examinations

— Authors —
N.A. Khan
Pramila Pandey
Md. Shamim
Deepti Srivastava

Daya Publishing House®
A Division of
Astral International Pvt. Ltd.
New Delhi – 110 002

Publisher's Note:

Every possible effort has been made to ensure that the information contained in this book is accurate at the time of going to press, and the publisher and author cannot accept responsibility for any errors or omissions, however caused. No responsibility for loss or damage occasioned to any person acting, or refraining from action, as a result of the material in this publication can be accepted by the editor, the publisher or the author. The Publisher is not associated with any product or vendor mentioned in the book. The contents of this work are intended to further general scientific research, understanding and discussion only. Readers should consult with a specialist where appropriate.

Every effort has been made to trace the owners of copyright material used in this book, if any. The author and the publisher will be grateful for any omission brought to their notice for acknowledgement in the future editions of the book.

Cataloging in Publication Data–DK
Courtesy: D.K. Agencies (P) Ltd. <docinfo@dkagencies.com>

Khan, N. A. (Nawaz Ahmad), author.

Question bank of biochemistry : for ready reference to the students, teachers and researchers, civil service examinations (state and central), NET, SET, Ph.D. and allied examinations / authors, N.A. Khan, Pramila Pandey, Md. Shamim, Deepti Srivastava.

pages cm
ISBN 9789390384433 (HB)

1. Biochemistry–Examinations, questions, etc. I. Pandey, Pramila, author. II. Shamim, Md. (Assistant professor of biotechnology), author. III. Srivastava, Deepti, author. IV. Title.

DDC 572.076 23

Published by : **Daya Publishing House®**
A Division of
Astral International Pvt. Ltd.
– ISO 9001:2015 Certified Company –
4736/23, Ansari Road, Darya Ganj
New Delhi-110 002
Ph. 011-43549197, 23278134
E-mail: info@astralint.com
Website: www.astralint.com

Preface

The first edition of the "Question Bank of Biochemistry" will primarily be helpful for fresh graduates and post-graduate of Biochemistry, Microbiology, Biotechnology, Immunology and allied streams who can prepare themselves for both written as well as oral examinations.

Multiple type questions are asked in almost all written competitions conducted by various government or private organization either for admission or recruitment.

This book has been presented with the objective of providing a large selection of questions in all major aspects of Biochemistry, Microbiology and Biotechnology, Immunology and answer in the respective stream.

The book contains about 2064 questions on various aspects. We are very grateful to Vice-Chancellor of N.D. University of Agriculture & Technology, Kumarganj, Faizabad for having given us the opportunity to write the book. We would like to thanks to our colleagues in the Department. We would like to express my thanks to Anil Mittal (Director) and Dr. B.B. Singh and staff of Astral International Pvt. Ltd. for their constant willing help.

The authors will greatly appreciate knowing reader's views or suggestions for any further improvement of this book.

N.A. Khan

Parmila Pandey

Md. Shamim

Deepti Srivastava

Contents

Chapter 1
Plant Structure

1. **Which part of a plant contains the male sex cell?**
   (a) Ova (b) Style
   (c) Stamen (d) Pollen

2. **A cell without cell wall is called**
   (a) Apoplast (b) Protoplast
   (c) Symplast (d) None of these

3. **Both plant and animal cell possess**
   (a) Cell wall (b) Mitochondria
   (c) Central vacuoles (d) Chloroplast

4. **Water content of active protoplasm is**
   (a) 10 per cent (b) 40 per cent
   (c) 70 per cent (d) 90 per cent

5. **Cellular organelles are embedded in the**
   (a) Endoplasmic reticulum (b) Cristae
   (c) Cytosol (d) Microtubules

6. **The fluid matrix of a cell is called the**
   (a) Nucleus (b) Cytosol
   (c) Cytoskeleton (d) Endoplasmic reticulum

7. **The cell membrane is made up of**
   (a) Lipoproteins (b) Cellulose
   (c) Phospholipids (d) Phosphoproteins

8. **Tonoplast is a membrane around**
   (a) Cytoplasm (b) Vacuole
   (c) Nucleus (d) Mitochondria

9. **Specialized type of peroxisome and the site of glyoxylate pathway in certain plants is known as**
   (a) Gly-peroxisome
   (b) Lysosome
   (c) Glyoxysome
   (d) None of these

10. **The cellular organelle associated with photosynthesis is the**
   (a) Golgi complex
   (b) Mitochondrion
   (c) Lysosome
   (d) Chloroplast

11. **The cellular organelle associated with secretion is the**
   (a) Golgi complex
   (b) Mitochondrion
   (c) Ribosome
   (d) Lysosome

12. **Chemical energy is supplied to eukaryotic cells by**
   (a) Chloroplasts and golgi complexes
   (b) Mitochondria and ribosomes
   (c) Mitochondria only
   (d) Mitochondria and chloroplasts

13. **The element neon (Ne) has eight electrons in its outermost electron shell. How many covalent bonds will Ne readily form?**
   (a) None
   (b) One
   (c) Two
   (d) Four

14. **Which of the following elements is likely to form the least polar covalent bond with hydrogen?**
   (a) Nitrogen
   (b) Oxygen
   (c) Carbon
   (d) Phosphorus

15. **If the ester bonds of a triacylglycerol molecule's are broken then the kind of molecule, which would be soluble in water, is**
   (a) Fatty acid
   (b) Steroid
   (c) Glycogen
   (d) Glycerol

16. **Which of the following functional groups would make a carbon-based compound the least polar?**
   (a) Phosphate
   (b) Methyl
   (c) Carboxyl
   (d) Amino

17. **If the ends of the following polysaccharide are pulled, which one would stretch the most?**
   (a) Glycogen
   (b) Starch
   (c) Cellulose
   (d) None of these

18. "The universe tends towards maximum disorder" is stated by

(a) First law of thermodynamics

(b) Second law of thermodynamics

(c) Third law of thermodynamics

(d) None of the above

19. Cellular metabolism is an example of

(a) Equilibrium metabolism

(b) Steady-state metabolism

(c) A series of reactions occurring under standard conditions

(d) A series of reactions that defy the second law of thermodynamics

20. Any system that is not at equilibrium

(a) Is thermodynamically unstable, although it may be kinetically stable

(b) Is kinetically unstable, although it may be thermodynamically stable

(c) Is rushing toward equilibrium at a very rapid rate

(d) Requires an enzyme to reach equilibrium

21. Which of the following observations is not used as evidence to support the concept of endosymbiotic origin of chloroplasts and mitochondria?

(a) Both have their own DNA

(b) Both have their own ribosomes

(c) Both strongly resemble prokaryotes, especially in size

(d) Both can live and function independently of the cell

22. The mitochondria were known in the nineteenth century to be osmotically active on the basis of evidence that

(a) The mitochondrial matrix is hypotonic to the cellular cytoplasm

(b) The mitochondrial matrix is hypertonic to the cellular cytoplasm

(c) Mitochondria were derived from a symbiotic bacterium

(d) Mitochondria are surrounded by a semi permeable membrane

23. Which cell type is likely to have the most mitochondria?

(a) Fast-twitch muscle

(b) Slow-twitch muscle

(c) Liver cells

(d) Adipose cells

24. The composition of the inner mitochondrial membrane is most like that of

(a) The outer mitochondrial membrane

(b) The cell's plasma membrane

(c) Some bacterial plasma membranes

(d) The nuclear membrane.

25. Which of the following statements about the outer mitochondrial membrane is not true?

(a) The outer membrane is impermeable to hydrogen ions

(b) The outer membrane is highly permeable to substances of small molecular weight

(c) The outer membrane is about 50 per cent lipid and 50 per cent protein by weight

(d) The outer membrane contains porins

26. Which of the following can be found as a part of the mitochondrial matrix?

(a) Ribosomes (b) DNA

(c) Enzymes (d) All of these

27. Which of the following experimental results does not support Mitchell's chemiosmosis theory?

(a) Electron transport in isolated mitochondria was shown to result in acidification of the medium

(b) Addition of dinitrophenol to isolated mitochondria was shown to inhibit electron transport, but had no effect on ATP synthesis

(c) Addition of dinitrophenol to isolated mitochondria during electron transport was shown to inhibit acidification of the medium

(d) An artificial proton gradient across the inner mitochondrial membrane drives ATP synthesis in the absence of electron transport

28. Mitochondria can be expected most numerous in

(a) Green cells (b) Red blood cells

(c) Muscle cells (d) None of these

29. Which of the following statements about mitochondrial proteins is true?

(a) All mitochondrial proteins are coded for and synthesized in the mitochondria

(b) Some mitochondrial proteins are coded for and synthesized in the mitochondria and others are synthesized in nucleus

(c) All mitochondrial proteins are imported from the cytoplasm

(d) Mitochondrial proteins arise from other mitochondrial proteins

30. Why do some redox reactions in cells result in the transfer of electrons from a reductant with a higher standard redox potential to an oxidant with a lower standard redox potential?

(a) Redox potentials are defined under standard conditions, and cellular conditions are typically not standard conditions

(b) The rules governing oxidation and reduction apply only *in vitro*, and not *in vivo*

(c) Electrons always go from reductants with high redox potentials to oxidants with low redox potentials

(d) None of the above

31. What is the source of free energy (ΔG) for moving protons out of mitochondria against their concentration and electrical gradients?

(a) Glycolysis

(b) Creatine phosphate

(c) The redox reactions of electron transport

(d) ATP

32. Which of the following is not an electron carrier class in the electron transport chain?

(a) Flavoproteins (b) Cytochromes

(c) Iron - sulfur proteins (d) Cytochrome C oxidase

33. If complex III were incorporated into an artificial lipid vesicle in order to demonstrate it's proton translocating ability in isolation, which of the following would be an appropriate electron donor?

(a) Cytochrome C red (b) Cytochrome C peroxidase

(c) Ubiquinol (UQH_2) (d) Cytochrome C oxidase

34. Which molecule serves as a carrier of fatty acids in mitochondria?

(a) Acetyl-CoA (b) Carnitine

(c) Dolichol (d) Malonyl-CoA

35. Which is not true about a photon?

(a) It is a packet of light energy

(b) The shorter the wavelength, the greater the energy of the photons

(c) It is trapped by photosynthetic unit

(d) It donates electron to reduce carbon dioxide to glucose

36. Lysosomes are associated with

(a) Photosynthesis (b) Respiration

(c) Storage (d) Digestion

37. In plant cells, which of the following is not a function of the large central vacuoles of plant cells?

(a) Storage of food (b) Support

(c) Contractile regulation of water content (d) Waste storage

Answers

1	(c)	11	(a)	21	(d)	31	(c)
2	(b)	12	(d)	22	(d)	32	(d)
3	(b)	13	(a)	23	(b)	33	(c)
4	(d)	14	(c)	24	(c)	34	(b)
5	(c)	15	(d)	25	(a)	35	(d)
6	(b)	16	(b)	26	(d)	36	(d)
7	(a)	17	(b)	27	(b)	37	(c)
8	(b)	18	(b)	28	(c)		
9	(c)	19	(b)	29	(b)		
10	(d)	20	(a)	30	(a)		

Chapter 2
Acid Base Balance

1. **The pH of gastric juice of infants is**
   (a) 5.0
   (b) 4.0
   (c) 5.0
   (d) 4.50

2. **Major buffering system in blood is**
   (a) Protein and H protein
   (b) K_2HPO_4 and KH_2PO_4
   (c) $NaHCO_3$ and H_2CO_3
   (d) Haemoglobin and H Haemoglobin

3. **In the reaction HADH$^+$ + A$^-$, the conjugate acid and conjugate base are**
   (a) HA and H^+
   (b) HA and H^-
   (c) $H^+ + A^-$
   (d) $A^+$and H^+

4. **The pH of a buffer is determined by pH= pKa + log [salt]/[acid] and the name of this equation is**
   (a) Gibbs-Donnam
   (b) Henderson-Joules
   (c) Henderson-Hasselbach
   (d) All of the above

5. **The sedimentation velocity of a particle depends on**
   (a) Its mass only
   (b) Mass and density
   (c) Shape of particle
   (d) All of the above

6. **During diffusion, the movement of solute particle occurs as**
   (a) From lower concentration to higher
   (b) From higher concentration to lower
   (c) All of the above
   (d) None of the above

7. **Vant Hoff's law is concerned with**
   (a) Strong electrolytes
   (b) Ionic solutions
   (c) Osmotic pressure
   (d) Weak electrolytes

8. **In dialysis protein molecules are separated on the basis of**
   (a) Molecular size
   (b) Net molecular charge
   (c) Dialysis coefficient
   (d) Pressure across semi permeable membrane

9. **The osmotic pressure of a solution increase with the rise in**
   (a) Humidity
   (b) Temperature
   (c) Cold
   (d) All of the above

10. **Adsorption decrease with rise in**
   (a) Temperature
   (b) Humidity
   (c) Cold
   (d) Dryness

11. **The sedimentation coefficient "S" is defined as**
   (a) The velocity divided by the centrifugal force
   (b) The velocity divided by centrifugal field
   (c) The centrifugal force divided by the effective mass of the particle
   (d) The centrifugal field divided by the velocity

12. **The molecular weight of a solute particle is**
   (a) Inversely proportional to osmotic pressure
   (b) Directly proportional to osmotic pressure
   (c) Independent of osmotic pressure
   (d) Inversely proportional to square of osmotic pressure

13. **The viscosity of a solution increase due to the pressure of**
   (a) Small sized particle
   (b) Soluble particles
   (c) Suspended particle
   (d) All of the above

14. **Surface tension of solution is increased by**
   (a) Acetic acid
   (b) Concentrated H_2SO_4
   (c) Bile salts
   (d) Bile acid

15. **The phenomenon of osmosis is opposite to**
   (a) Adsorption
   (b) Effusion
   (c) Diffusion
   (d) Dialysis

16. In case of non-homogenous solution diffusion is expressed as ds/dt=DA.dc/dx by

(a) Ficks law (b) Peterson law
(c) Faraday's law (d) Dicks law

17. The average pH of urine is

(a) 5.6 (b) 6.0
(c) 6.4 (d) 6.8

18. The osmotic pressure of a solution relating to solute molecule depends on the

(a) Size (b) Shape
(c) Number (d) Volume

19. If a cell immersed in a concentrated solution, it follws the phenomenon of

(a) Turger pressure (b) Plasmolysis
(c) Hemolysis (d) Paralysis

20. The intracellular fluid of red cells and the red cell membrane in 0.92 per cent NaCl solution are

(a) Osmosis (b) Adsorption
(c) Diffusion (d) Absorption

21. The Purgative action of Epsom ($MgSO_4$) salt follows

(a) Osmosis (b) Diffusion
(c) Effusion (d) Imbibition

22. Hemolysis is caused by the dilution of RBC by

(a) Osmosis (b) Diffusion
(c) Effusion (d) Imbibition

23. The process of adsorption is applied in the purification of

(a) Enzymes (b) Vitamin
(c) Coenzymes (d) Hormones

24. Bile salt make emulsion with fat for the action of

(a) Amylose (b) Lipase
(c) Pepsin (d) Trypsin

25. The size of each colloidal particle in nm is

(a) 4 to 40 (b) 6 to 60
(c) 8 to 80 (d) 10 to 100

26. The sperm colloidal protein particles may be precipitated by the addition of large amount of

(a) Ammonium sulphate (b) Calcium sulphate
(c) Barium sulphate (d) Magnesium sulphate

27. Water is not expelled by squeezing in

(a) Imbibition (b) Precipitation
(c) Combination (d) Dilution

28. Fatty acids can be transported into and out of mitochondria through

(a) Active transport (b) Passive diffusion
(c) Simple diffusion (d) Non facilitated transport

29. The absorption of intact protein from the gut in the fetal and new born animal takes place by

(a) Pinocytosis (b) Passive diffusion
(c) Simple diffusion (d) Active transport

Answers

1	(c)	9	(b)	17	(b)	25	(d)
2	(c)	10	(a)	18	(c)	26	(a)
3	(b)	11	(b)	19	(b)	27	(a)
4	(c)	12	(a)	20	(c)	28	(b)
5	(d)	13	(c)	21	(a)	29	(a)
6	(b)	14	(b)	22	(a)		
7	(c)	15	(c)	23	(a)		
8	(a)	16	(a)	24	(b)		

Chapter 3
Acid Base

1. **A person was admitted in a coma. Analysis of the arterial blood gave the following values: PCO_2 16 mm Hg, HCO_3- 5 mmol/l and pH 7.1. What is the underlying acid-base disorder?**
   (a) Metabolic Acidosis (b) Metabolic Alkalosis
   (c) Respiratory Acidosis (d) Respiratory Alkalosis

2. **In a man undergoing surgery, it was necessary to aspirate the contents of the upper gastrointestinal tract. After surgery, the following values were obtained from an arterial blood sample: pH 7.55, PCO_2 52 mm Hg and HCO_3- 40 mmol/l. What is the underlying disorder?**
   (a) Metabolic Acidosis (b) Metabolic Alkalosis
   (c) Respiratory Acidosis (d) Respiratory Alkalosis

3. **A young woman is found comatose, having taken an unknown number of sleeping pills an unknown time before. An arterial blood sample yields the following values: pH – 6.90, HCO_3-13 meq/liter, $PaCO_2$ 68 mmHg. This patient's acid-base status is most accurately described as**
   (a) Uncompensated metabolic acidosis
   (b) Uncompensated respiratory acidosis
   (c) Simultaneous respiratory and metabolic acidosis
   (d) Respiratory acidosis with partial renal compensation

4. **A student is nervous for a big exam and is breathing rapidly, what do you expect out of the following**
   (a) Metabolic Acidosis (b) Metabolic Alkalosis
   (c) Respiratory Acidosis (d) Respiratory Alkalosis

5. **A 45-year-old female with renal failure, missed her dialysis and was feeling sick, what could be the reason ?**
   (a) Metabolic Acidosis (b) Metabolic Alkalosis
   (c) Respiratory Acidosis (d) Respiratory Alkalosis

6. **An 80-year-old man had a bad cold. After two weeks he said, "It went in to my chest, I am feeling tightness in my chest, I am coughing, suffocated and unable to breathe!" What could be the possible reason?**
   (a) Metabolic Acidosis (b) Metabolic Alkalosis
   (c) Respiratory Acidosis (d) Respiratory Alkalosis

7. **A post operative surgical patient had a naso gastric tube in for three days. The nurse caring for the patient stated that there was much drainage from the tube that is why she felt so sick. What could be the reason?**
   (a) Metabolic Acidosis (b) Metabolic Alkalosis
   (c) Respiratory Acidosis (d) Respiratory Alkalosis

8. **The pH of the body fluids is stabilized by buffer systems. Which of the following compounds is the most effective buffer system at physiological pH?**
   (a) Bicarbonate buffer (b) Phosphate buffer
   (c) Protein buffer (d) All of the above

9. **Which of the following laboratory results below indicates compensated metabolic alkalosis?**
   (a) Low p CO_2, normal bicarbonate and, high pH
   (b) Low p CO_2, low bicarbonate, low pH
   (c) High p CO_2, normal bicarbonate and, low pH
   (d) High pCO_2, high bicarbonate and High pH

10. **The greatest buffering capacity at physiological p H would be provided by a protein rich in which of the following amino acids?**
    (a) Lysine (b) Histidine
    (c) Aspartic acid (d) Leucine

11. **Which of the following is most appropriate for a female suffering from Insulin dependent diabetes mellitus with a pH of 7.2, HCO_3-17 mmol/L and pCO2-20 mm HG**
    (a) Metabolic Acidosis (b) Metabolic Alkalosis
    (c) Respiratory Acidosis (d) Respiratory Alkalosis

12. **Causes of metabolic alkalosis include all the following except.**
    (a) Mineralocorticoid deficiency. (b) Hypokalemia
    (c) Thiazide diuretic therapy. (d) Recurrent vomiting.

13. **Renal Glutaminase activity is increased in**
    (a) Metabolic acidosis (b) Respiratory Acidosis
    (c) Both of the above (d) None of the above

14. Causes of lactic acidosis include all except

(a) Acute Myocardial infarction
(b) Hypoxia
(c) Circulatory failure
(d) Infections

15. Which out of the following conditions will not cause respiratory alkalosis?

(a) Fever
(b) Anxiety
(c) Laryngeal obstruction
(d) Salicylate toxicity

16. All are true about metabolic alkalosis except one

(a) Associated with hyperkalemia
(b) Associated with decreased ionic calcium concentration
(c) Can be caused due to Primary hyperaldosteronism
(d) Can be caused due to Renin secreting tumor

17. Choose the incorrect statement out of the following

(a) Deoxy haemoglobin is a weak base
(b) Oxyhaemoglobin is a relatively strong acid
(c) The buffering capacity of haemoglobin is lesser than plasma protein
(d) The buffering capacity of Haemoglobin is due to histidine residues.

18. Carbonic anhydrase is present at all places except

(a) Gastric parietal cells
(b) Red blood cells
(c) Renal tubular cells
(d) Plasma

19. All are true for renal handling of acids in metabolic acidosis except

(a) Hydrogen ion secretion is increased
(b) Bicarbonate reabsorption is decreased
(c) Urinary acidity is increased
(d) Urinary ammonia is increased.

20. Choose the incorrect statement about anion gap out of the following

(a) In lactic acidosis anion gap is increased
(b) Anion gap is decreased in Hypercalcemia
(c) Anion gap is decreased in Lithium toxicity
(d) Anion gap is decreased in ketoacidosis

21. Excessive citrate in transfused blood can cause which of the following abnormalities?

(a) Metabolic alkalosis
(b) Metabolic acidosis
(c) Respiratory alkalosis
(d) Respiratory acidosis

Fill in the Blanks

1. The largest compartment of body fluids is the __________ compartment.
2. Water makes up __________ per cent of the body's weight in a healthy adult.
3. The main extracellular anion is __________.
4. The main intracellular cation is __________.
5. ADH causes the renal tubules to retain __________.
6. Potassium secretion in the renal tubules is regulated by __________.
7. Normal plasma pH is __________.

Answers

1	(a)	7	(b)	13	(c)	19	(b)
2	(b)	8	(a)	14	(d)	20	(d)
3	(c)	9	(d)	15	(c)	21	(a)
4	(d)	10	(b)	16	(a)		
5	(a)	11	(a)	17	(c)		
6	(c)	12	(a)	18	(d)		

Fill in the Blanks

1. Intracellular
2. 60
3. Chloride
4. Potassium
5. Water
6. Aldosterone
7. 7.4

Chapter 4
Biological Oxidation

1. **Membrane potential and the proton gradient**
   (a) Are both required to make ATP
   (b) Are sufficient, separately, to make ATP from ADP + Pi
   (c) Reinforce one another when respiratory inhibitors are present
   (d) Cancel one another when uncouplers are present

2. **The three identical b subunits of the Fi complex during ATP synthesis have**
   (a) Different affinities for ATP but not for ADP
   (b) Different affinities for ADP but not for ATP
   (c) Different affinities for ATP and for ADP
   (d) Similar affinities for ADP and ATP

3. **Long-chain fatty acids are oxidized step-wise in one carbon units starting from the**
   (a) Carboxyl end
   (b) Aliphatic end
   (c) Both (a) and (b)
   (d) None of these

4. **The irreversibility of the thiokinase reactions (formation of initial acyl-CoA)**
   (a) Make this activation reaction the committed step on the pathway
   (b) Is due to the subsequent hydrolysis of the product
   (c) Applies only to even-chain fatty acids
   (d) Both (a) and (b)

5. **Where the acyl-CoA formed in the cytosol is transported for oxidation?**
   (a) Mitochondrial matrix
   (b) Microsomes
   (c) Endoplasmic reticulum
   (d) Remains in cytosol

6. **The transport of acyl-CoA for oxidation using a shuttle involves formation of the intermediate**
   (a) 3 acetyl-CoA
   (b) Acyl-coenzyme A
   (c) Acyl-carnitine
   (d) None of these

7. **Each cycle of a-oxidation produces**
   (a) I $FADH_2$, I NAD^+, and 1 acetyl-CoA
   (b) 1 $FADH_2$, I NADH and 1 acetyl-CoA
   (c) $FADH_2$, I NADH and 2 CO_2 molecules
   (d) I FAD, 1 NAD^+ and 2 CO_2 molecules

8. **How many molecules of acetyl-CoA are produced in oxidation of palmitic acid (C_{16}), which involves seven rounds of oxidation?**
   (a) 6
   (b) 7
   (c) 8
   (d) 9

9. **The maximum energy per gram on oxidization is yielded from**
   (a) Fat
   (b) Protein
   (c) Glycogen
   (d) Starch

10. **The oxidation of methanol (wood alcohol) in human retina tissue leads directly to the formation of**
    (a) Formaldehyde
    (b) Sugars
    (c) CO_2
    (d) None of these

11. **The oxidation of methanol (wood alcohol) in human retina tissue indirectly leads to**
    (a) Pressure builds up
    (b) Colour blindness
    (c) Blindness
    (d) All of these

Answers

1	(a)	4	(d)	7	(b)	10	(a)
2	(c)	5	(a)	8	(c)	11	(c)
3	(a)	6	(c)	9	(a)		

Chapter 5
Oxidative Phosphorylation Electron Transport

1. **A biological redox reaction always involves**
   (a) An oxidizing agent
   (b) A gain of electrons
   (c) A reducing agent
   (d) All of these

2. **Which of the following is not a feature of oxidative phosphorylation**
   (a) Direct transfer of phosphate from a substrate molecule to ADP
   (b) An electrochemical gradient across the inner mitochondrial membrane
   (c) A membrane bound ATP synthase
   (d) A protonmotive force

3. **Which of the following is not a significant biological oxidizing agent?**
   (a) FAD
   (b) Fe^{3+}
   (c) O_2
   (d) NAD^+

4. **During electron transport, protons are pumped out of the mitochondrion at each of the major sites except for**
   (a) Complex I
   (b) Complex II
   (c) Complex III
   (d) Complex IV

5. **Coenzyme Q is involved in electron transport as**
   (a) Directly to O_2
   (b) A water-soluble electron donor
   (c) Covalently attached cytochrome cofactor
   (d) A lipid-soluble electron carrier

6. **How many CO_2 molecules are exhaled for each O_2 molecule utilized in cellular respiration?**
   (a) 1
   (b) 3
   (c) 6
   (d) 12

7. **Which of the following is correct sequence of processes in the oxidation of glucose?**
   (a) Krebs cycle - glycolysis - electron transport
   (b) Glycolysis - Krebs cycle - eletron transport
   (c) Electron transport - Krebs cycle - glycolysis
   (d) Krebs cycle - electron transport - glycolysis

8. **The complete oxidation of glucose yields usable energy in the form of**
   (a) $FADH_2$ (b) Coenzyme A
   (c) ATP (d) Pyruvic acid

9. **During glycolysis, electrons removed from glucose are passed to**
   (a) FAD (b) NAD^+
   (c) Acetyl CoA (d) Pyruvic acid

10. **In electron transport, electrons ultimately pass to**
    (a) ADP (b) Cytochrome b
    (c) Oxygen (d) None of these

11. **Lactic acid is produced by human muscles during strenuous exercise because of lack of**
    (a) Oxygen (b) NAD^+
    (c) Glucose (d) ADP and P_i

12. **The aerobic breakdown of glucose known as respiration involves**
    (a) Electron transport phosphorylation (b) Glycolysis
    (c) Krebs Cycle (d) All of the above

13. **In aerobic respiration, the compound that enters a mitochondrion is**
    (a) Acetyl CoA (b) Pyruvate
    (c) Phosphoglyceraldehyde (d) Oxaloacetate

14. **FAD is reduced to $FADH_2$ during**
    (a) Electron transport phosphorylation (b) Lactate fermentation
    (c) Krebs cycle (d) Glycolysis

15. **The carbon dioxide is primary a product of**
    (a) Krebs cycle (b) Glycolysis
    (c) Electron transport phosphorylation (d) Lactate fermentation.

16. **What happens after glycolysis when oxygen is available as an electron acceptor?**
    (a) Pyruvate is formed (b) NADH is produced
    (c) Fermentation (d) Oxidative phosphorylation

Answers

1	(d)	5	(d)	9	(b)	13	(b)
2	(a)	6	(a)	10	(c)	14	(c)
3	(b)	7	(c)	11	(a)	15	(a)
4	(b)	8	(c)	12	(d)	16	(b)

Chapter 6
Cell Biology

1. **A drug which prevents uric acid synthesis by inhibiting the enzyme xanthine oxidase is**
   (a) Aspirin (b) Allopurinol
   (c) Colchicine (d) Probenecid
2. **Which of the following is required for crystallization and storage of the hormone insulin?**
   (a) Mn^{++} (b) Mg^{++}
   (c) Ca^{++} (d) Zn^{++}
3. **Oxidation of which substance in the body yields the most calories**
   (a) Glucose (b) Glycogen
   (c) Protein (d) Lipids
4. **Milk is deficient in which vitamins?**
   (a) Vitamin C (b) Vitamin A
   (c) Vitamin B_2 (d) Vitamin K
5. **Milk is deficient of which mineral?**
   (a) Phosphorus (b) Sodium
   (c) Iron (d) Potassium
6. **Synthesis of prostaglandinsis is inhibited by**
   (a) Aspirin (b) Arsenic
   (c) Fluoride (d) Cyanide
7. **HDL is synthesized and secreted from**
   (a) Pancreas (b) Liver
   (c) Kidney (d) Muscle

8. Which are the cholesterol esters that enter cells through the receptor-mediated endocytosis of lipoproteins hydrolyzed?

(a) Endoplasmic reticulum (b) Lysosomes
(c) Plasma membrane receptor (d) Mitochondria

9. Which of the following phospholipids is localized to a greater extent in the outer leaflet of the membrane lipid bilayer?

(a) Choline phosphoglycerides (b) Inositol phosphoglycerides
(c) Ethanolamine phosphoglycerides (d) Serine phosphoglycerides

10. All the following processes occur rapidly in the membrane lipid bilayer except

(a) Flexing of fatty acyl chains
(b) Lateral diffusion of phospholipids
(c) Transbilayer diffusion of phopholipids
(d) Rotation of phospholipids around their long axes

11. Which of the following statement is correct about membrane cholesterol?

(a) The hydroxyl group is located near the centre of the lipid layer
(b) Most of the cholesterol is in the form of a cholesterol ester
(c) The steroid nucleus form forms a rigid, planar structure
(d) The hydrocarbon chain of cholesterol projects into the extracellular fluid

12. Which one is the heaviest particulate component of the cell?

(a) Nucleus (b) Mitochondria
(c) Cytoplasm (d) Golgi apparatus

13. Which one is the largest particulate of the cytoplasm?

(a) Lysosomes (b) Mitochondria
(c) Golgi apparatus (d) Entoplasmic reticulum

14. The degradative Processess are categorized under the heading of

(a) Anabolism (b) Catabolism
(c) Metabolism (d) None of the above

15. The exchange of material takes place

(a) Only by diffusion (b) Only by active transport
(c) Only by pinocytosis (d) All of these

16. The average pH of Urine is

(a) 7.0 (b) 6.0
(c) 8.0 (d) 0.0

17. The pH of blood is 7.4 when the ratio between H_2CO_3 and $NaHCO_3$ is

(a) 1: 10 (b) 1: 20

(c) 1: 25 (d) 1: 30

18. The phenomenon of osmosis is opposite to that of

(a) Diffusion (b) Effusion

(c) Affusion (d) Coagulation

19. The surface tension in intestinal lumen between fat droplets and aqueous medium is decreased by

(a) Bile Salts (b) Bile acids

(c) Conc. H_2SO_4 (d) Acetic acid

20. Which of the following is located in the mitochondria?

(a) Cytochrome oxidase (b) Succinate dehydrogenase

(c) Dihydrolipoyl dehydrogenase (c) All of these

21. The most active site of protein synthesis is the

(a) Nucleus (b) Ribosome

(c) Mitochondrion (d) Cell sap

22. The fatty acids can be transported into and out of mitochondria through

(a) Active transport (b) Facilitated transfer

(c) Non-facilitated transfer (d) None of these

23. Mitochondrial DNA is

(a) Circular double stranded (b) Circular single stranded

(c) Linear double helix (d) None of these

24. The absorption of intact protein from the gut in the foetal and newborn animals takes place by

(a) Pinocytosis (b) Passive diffusion

(c) Simple diffusion (d) Active transport

25. The cellular organelles called "suicide bags" are

(a) Lysosomes (b) Ribosomes

(c) Nucleolus (d) Golgi's bodies

26. From the biological viewpoint, solutions can be grouped into

(a) Isotonic solution (b) Hypotonic solution

(c) Hypertonic solution (d) All of these

27. Bulk transport across cell membrane is accomplished by

(a) Phagocytosis (b) Pinocytosis

(c) Extrusion (d) All of these

28. The ability of the cell membrane to act as a selective barrier depends upon

(a) The lipid composition of the membrane
(b) The pores which allows small molecules
(c) The special mediated transport systems
(d) All of these

29. Carrier protein can

(a) Transport more than one substance
(b) Perform all of these functions
(c) Exchange one substance to another
(d) Transport only one substance

30. A lipid bilayer is permeable to

(a) Urea
(b) Fructose
(c) Glucose
(d) Potassium

31. The Golgi complex

(a) Synthesizes proteins
(b) Produces ATP
(c) Provides a pathway for transporting chemicals
(d) Forms glycoproteins

32. The following points about microfilaments are true except

(a) They form cytoskeleton with microtubules
(b) They provide support and shape
(c) They form intracellular conducting channels
(d) They are involved in muscle cell contraction

33. The following substances are cell inclusions except

(a) Melanin
(b) Glycogen
(c) Lipids
(d) Centrosome

34. Fatty acids can be transported into and out of cell membrane by

(a) Active transport
(b) Facilitated transport
(c) Diffusion
(d) Osmosis

35. Enzymes catalyzing electron transport are present mainly in the

(a) Ribosomes
(b) Endoplasmic reticulum
(c) Inner mitochondrial membrane
(d) Lysosomes

36. Mature erythrocytes do not contain

(a) Glycolytic enzymes
(b) HMP shunt enzymes
(c) Pyridine nucleotide
(d) ATP

37. In mammalian cells rRNA is produced mainly in the

(a) Endoplasmic reticulum
(b) Ribosome
(c) Nucleolus
(d) Nucleus

38. Genetic information of nuclear DNA is transmitted to the site of protein synthesis by

(a) *r*RNA
(b) *m*RNA
(c) *t*RNA
(d) Polysomes

39. The power house of the cell is

(a) Nucleus
(b) Cell membrane
(c) Mitochondria
(d) Lysosomes

40. The digestive enzymes of cellular compounds are confined to

(a) Lysosomes
(b) Ribosomes
(c) Peroxisomes
(d) Polysomes

Answers

1	(b)	11	(c)	21	(b)	31	(d)
2	(d)	12	(a)	22	(b)	32	(c)
3	(d)	13	(b)	23	(a)	33	(d)
4	(a)	14	(b)	24	(a)	34	(b)
5	(c)	15	(d)	25	(a)	35	(c)
6	(a)	16	(b)	26	(d)	36	(c)
7	(b)	17	(b)	27	(d)	37	(c)
8	(b)	18	(a)	28	(d)	38	(d)
9	(a)	19	(a)	29	(b)	39	(c)
10	(c)	20	(d)	30	(a)	40	(a)

Chapter 7

Photosynthesis and Respiration

1. **In the initial step of photosynthesis, sunlight energizes the electron pair of**
   (a) Adenosine triphosphate (ATP) (b) Chlorophyll pigments
   (c) Water (d) Carbon dioxide

2. **As a result of the photosynthetic process, which product is formed?**
   (a) Oxygen (b) Water
   (c) Carbon dioxide (d) Both (a) and (b)

3. **In cells having organelles, the steps of the Krebs cycle and the electron transport system occur in the**
   (a) Cell membrane (b) Mitochondria
   (c) Endoplasmic reticulum (d) None of these

4. **The breakdown of glucose occurs by the process known as**
   (a) Glycolysis (b) Fermentation
   (c) Anaerobic respiration (d) Krebs cycle

5. **A cyclic electron transport process is the characteristic of**
   (a) Photosynthesis (b) Methane oxidation
   (c) Sulfide oxidation (d) Methane production

6. **In oxygenic photosynthesis, the electron donor is**
   (a) Water (b) Oxygen
   (c) NADH (d) NADPH

7. **In the Calvin cycle, carbon dioxide is fixed in a reaction with the**
   (a) Ribulose diphosphate (b) Ribulose phosphate
   (c) Ribose tri phosphate (d) 3-phosphoglyceric acid

8. **Electron transport systems play a vital role in**
   (a) Calvin cycle
   (b) Photorespiration
   (c) Light-dependent reactions
   (d) All of these

9. **NADP is reduced to NADPH during**
   (a) Light dependent reactions
   (b) Photorespiration
   (c) Calvin cylcle
   (d) None of these

10. **Which one of the following is a product of both cyclic and noncyclic photophosphorylation?**
   (a) NADPH
   (b) O_2
   (c) ATP
   (d) Carbohydrate

11. **If the oxygen is labeled in CO_2 and provide this CO_2 to a plant, where it is expected to find this labeled oxygen after the plant had undergone photosynthesis?**
   (a) In the water used
   (b) In the NADPH
   (c) In the carbohydrate produced
   (d) IN the oxygen given off by the plant

12. **In noncyclic photophosphorylation, the ultimate acceptor of electrons that have been produced from the splitting of water is**
   (a) $NADP^+$
   (b) Chlorophyll *a*
   (c) Carbon dioxide
   (d) Chlorophyll *b*

13. **The followings are the products of the light reactions of photosynthesis except**
   (a) ATP
   (b) Oxygen
   (c) NADPH
   (d) Glucose

14. **In oxygenic photosynthesis, water is split in order to provide the**
   (a) Electrons needed to reduce P680
   (b) O_2 needed for the dark reactions
   (c) Electrons needed to reduce NADH
   (d) Electrons needed for cyclic photophosphorylation

15. **Carbon dioxide is reduced in**
   (a) Noncyclic photophosphorylation
   (b) The Calvin cycle
   (c) The light reactions
   (d) Both light and dark reactions

16. The end products of noncyclic photophosphorylation are

(a) O_2, ATP and NADPH

(b) Carbon dioxide, PGAL (phosphoglyceraldehyde), and H_2

(c) Water, ADP and NADP

(d) Carbon dioxide, ATP and water

17. Carbon fixation requires the expenditure ofATP molecules which is generated by

(a) Formation of glucose during the Calvin cycle

(b) Replenishment of chlorophyll

(c) ETS (electron transfer system) during the light reactions

(d) None of the above

18. The rate of photorespiration in most plants increases at higher temperatures. Some plants have evolved a somewhat round-about system to deal with this problem. This series of reactions is called

(a) ETS (electron transfer system in light reactions

(b) C_4 pathway

(c) Photosystem II

(d) Calvin cycle

19. In algae, photosynthesis takes place in

(a) Choloroplasts

(b) Cell membrane

(c) Mitochondria

(d) None of the above

20. What is the maximum absorption wavelength for photosystem I in green plants?

(a) 550 nm

(b) 600 nm

(c) 700 nm

(d) 750 nm

21. Which enzyme is involved in carbon-fixation reaction?

(a) NADP reductase

(b) Cytochrome reductase

(c) Ribulose bisphosphate carboxylase

(d) Glycerol kinase

22. The cytochrome c oxidase complex

(a) Accepts electrons from cyt C

(b) Donates four electrons to O_2

(c) Pumps protons out of the matrix space

(d) All of these

23. During the light-dependent reactions of photosynthesis, which of the following does not occur?

(a) Splitting of water
(b) Carbon dioxide fixation
(c) Release of oxygen
(d) Absorption of light energy by photosystems

24. Hydrogen (electron) acceptor in the light reactions is

(a) ADP (b) $NADP^+$
(c) NA D+ (d) FADH

25. Which of the following statements about energy metabolism is false?

(a) The energy that powers living systems ultimately comes from the sun
(b) All animals in some way rely on plants for their energy
(c) Plants provide the water and CO_2 that animals need to carry out respiration
(d) All eukaryotic organisms carry out respiration in the presence of O_2

26. Which of the following is the reduced form of a temporary electron carrier molecule?

(a) $FADH_2$ (b) ATP
(c) $NADP^+$ (d) CO_2

27. The vast majority of the molecules that act as energy carriers to power cellular activities are made in

(a) The nucleus
(b) The Golgi apparatus
(c) The cytosol
(d) The mitochondria and chloroplasts

28. Which of the following structures or processes are logically associated with chloroplasts?

(a) Plant cells (b) Chlorophyll
(c) Thylakoid membranes (d) All of these

29. Antenna complexes, electron transport chains, and carbon fixation are all found in

(a) Animal cells
(b) Bacterial cells
(c) Plant cells
(d) Association with the reactions of the citric acid cycle

30. The manufacture of ATP in both photosynthesis and respiration is made possible by

(a) The existence of a proton gradient across specific membranes

(b) The action of ATP synthase

(c) Energy from the movement of electrons

(d) All of the above

31. Rubisco (RuBP Carboxylase-oxygenase enzyme), glyceraldehyde 3-phosphate, and NADPH all play a role in

(a) The dark reactions of photosynthesis

(b) The breakdown of glucose into CO_2

(c) Cellular respiration when O_2 is present

(d) Alcohol fermentation

32. Which of the following represents a correct ordering of the events that occur during the respiration of glucose in the absence of O_2?

(a) Glycolysis; citric acid cycle; oxidative phosphorylation

(b) Glycolysis; oxidative phosphorylation; citric acid cycle

(c) Oxidative phosphorylation; citric acid cycle; glycolysis

(d) Glycolysis; fermentation

33. Glycolysis takes places in the ________ and produces ________ which in the presence of oxygen then enters the ________

(a) Cytosol; glucose; mitochondrion to complete fermentation

(b) Cytosol; pyruvate; mitochondrion to complete fermentation

(c) Cytosol; pyruvate; mitochondrion to complete cellular respiration

(d) Mitochondrion; pyruvate; chloroplast to complete photosynthesis

34. More ATP is manufactured during ________ than at any other time in all of cellular metabolism.

(a) Fermentation

(b) Glycolysis

(c) The light reactions of photosynthesis

(d) Oxidative phosphorylation

35. Where does the O_2 come from that is essential for the proper functioning of oxidative phosphorylation?

(a) Fermentation

(b) Light reactions of photosynthesis

(c) Dark reactions of photosynthesis

(d) Carbon fixation

36. What do NAD^+, NADP, and FAD^+ all have in common?

(a) They are reduced

(b) They have a full complement of electrons

(c) They are oxidized

(d) They are what is used during carbon fixation in photosynthesis

37. Which of the following serves as a reactant in photosynthesis and a product in cellular respiration?

(a) O_2
(b) CO_2
(c) Sunlight
(d) ATP

38. Where do the protons come from that make up the proton gradient used in the light reactions of photosynthesis?

(a) Glucose
(b) ATP
(c) H_2O
(d) NADPH

39. The electrons that are released by the splitting of water during photosynthesis ultimately end up in

(a) ATP
(b) O_2
(c) NADPH
(d) Rubisco

40. What process in cellular respiration is essentially the reverse of carbon fixation in photosynthesis?

(a) Glycolysis
(b) Citric acid cycle
(c) Oxidative phosphorylation
(d) Alcohol fermentation

41. What do coenzyme A, CO_2, oxaloacetate, and $FADH_2$ all have in common?

(a) They are part of the dark reactions of photosynthesis

(b) They are all components or products of the citric acid cycle

(c) They are part of the reactions of lactic acid fermentation

(d) They are all elements of oxidative phosphorylation

42. Assume the combined processes of photosynthesis and cellular respiration, the electrons that start as part of H_2O at the beginning of the light reactions end up attaching to

(a) O_2 to make new H_2O

(b) NADPH to make new glucose

(c) Pyruvate to make ethanol

(d) Electron transport carriers to make O_2

43. A eukaryotic cell that can carry out only fermentation instead of the complete aerobic respiration of glucose

(a) Produces less CO_2

(b) Is lacking in O_2

(c) Has mitochondria present

(d) All of these

44. Oxidative phosphorylation is to respiration as ________ to photosynthesis

(a) Carbon fixation

(b) Electron transport chain

(c) Light capture by chlorophyll

(d) Reduction of NADPH

Answers

1	(b)	12	(c)	23	(b)	34	(d)
2	(a)	13	(d)	24	(b)	35	(b)
3	(b)	14	(a)	25	(c)	36	(c)
4	(a)	15	(b)	26	(a)	37	(b)
5	(a)	16	(a)	27	(d)	38	(c)
6	(a)	17	(c)	28	(d)	39	(c)
7	(a)	18	(b)	29	(c)	40	(b)
8	(c)	19	(a)	30	(d)	41	(a)
9	(a)	20	(c)	31	(a)	42	(a)
10	(c)	21	(c)	32	(d)	43	(d)
11	(c)	22	(d)	33	(c)	44	(b)

Chapter 8
Carbohydrate Metabolism

1. **Metabolic reactions that break down complex molecules into smaller compounds, thereby releasing usable energy for the cell, are best described as**
   (a) Biosynthetic (b) Catabolic
   (c) Catalytic (d) Photosynthetic

2. **The ultimate source of energy that sustains living systems is**
   (a) Glucose (b) Oxygen
   (c) Sunlight (d) Carbon dioxide

3. **Which of the following is not a disaccharide?**
   (a) Amylose (b) Cellobiose
   (c) Lactose (d) None of these

4. **What is the cause of the genetic disease known as Galactosemia?**
   (a) Deficiency in lactase
   (b) Absence of galactose 1-P uridyl transferase
   (c) Absence of lactose synthetase
   (d) Non functioning of semnase

5. **What is the consensus N-glycosylation site in a protein sequence?**
   (a) Asn-Xaa-(Ser or Thr) (b) (Ser or Thr)-Asn-Ala
   (c) Thr-(Asn or Gln)-Ala (d) None of these

6. **Which of the following statements about the energy needs of cells is false?**
   (a) Without a continuous input of energy, cell disorder will increase
   (b) The laws of thermodynamics force cells to acquire energy
   (c) Many cellular reactions have an associated activation energy
   (d) The most usable energy for cells comes from the rapid combustion of glucose

7. **The production or break down of is often coupled with the metabolic reactions of biosynthesis and catabolism.**
   (a) Aspirin (b) DNA
   (c) ATP (d) CO_2

8. **The multistep pathways of metabolism are efficient because they**
   (a) Locate all of the enzymes for a pathway in the same place within the cell
   (b) Use the same substrate for all of the enzymes in the pathway
   (c) Use the same enzyme for all of the substrates in the pathway
   (d) Spread the enzymes for a pathway into several different organelles

9. **Which of the following is not involved in the biosynthesis of DNA?**
   (a) Energy from ATP (b) Mononucleotides
   (c) Carbonic anhydrase (d) Enzymes

10. **Which of the following would be considered a part of metabolism?**
   (a) Biosynthetic pathways that build DNA
   (b) Catabolic pathways that break down complex carbohydrates
   (c) The capture of light energy for use in making glucose
   (d) All of the above

11. **A common way that cells capture the energy released during the breakdown of large molecules is to add electrons to smaller, specialized molecules that can accept them. This process of electron acceptance is otherwise known as**
   (a) Biosynthesis (b) Metabolism
   (c) Reduction (d) Catalysis

12. **When living organisms are cooled below some critical body temperature, the metabolic reactions within their cells cease to function properly. This malfunction occurs because**
   (a) Their enzymes lose the proper three-dimensional shape
   (b) Enzyme active sites become permanently bound to substrates
   (c) The activation energy for the reaction is raised
   (d) There is insufficient molecular motion for substrates to interact

13. **What would be the molecular formula for a polymer made by linking ten glucose molecules together by dehydration synthesis, if molecular formula for glucose is $C_6H_{12}O_6$?**
   (a) $C_{60}H_{100}O_{50}$ (b) $C_{60}H_{120}O_{60}$
   (c) $C_{60}H_{102}O_{51}$ (d) $(C_6H_{12}O_6)_{10}$

14. Boat and chair conformations are found

(a) In pyranose sugars

(b) In any sugar without axial -OH groups

(c) In any sugar without equatorial -OH groups

(d) only in D-glucopyranose

Answers

1	(b)	5	(a)	9	(c)	13	(c)
2	(c)	6	(d)	10	(d)	14	(a)
3	(a)	7	(c)	11	(c)		
4	(b)	8	(a)	12	(d)		

Chapter 9
Carbohydrate

1. **The general formula of monosaccharides is**
   (a) CnH_2nOn (b) C_2nH_2On
   (c) CnH_2O_2n (d) CnH_2nO_2n
2. **The general formula of polysaccharides is**
   (a) $(C_6H_{10}O_5)n$ (b) $(C_6H_{12}O_5)n$
   (c) $(C_6H_{10}O_6)n$ (d) $(C_6H_{10}O_6)n$
3. **The aldose sugar is**
   (a) Glycerose (b) Ribulose
   (c) Erythrulose (d) Dihydoxyacetone
4. **A triose sugar is**
   (a) Glycerose (b) Ribose
   (c) Erythrose (d) Fructose
5. **A pentose sugar is**
   (a) Dihydroxyacetone (b) Ribulose
   (c) Erythrose (d) Glucose
6. **The pentose sugar present mainly in the heart muscle is**
   (a) Lyxose (b) Ribose
   (c) Arabinose (d) Xylose
7. **Polysaccharides are**
   (a) Polymers (b) Acids
   (c) Proteins (d) Oils
8. **The number of isomers of glucose is**
   (a) 2 (b) 4
   (c) 8 (d) 16

9. Two sugars which differ from one another only in configuration around a single carbon atom are termed

(a) Epimers (b) Anomers
(c) Optical isomers (d) Stereoisomers

10. Isomers differing as a result of variations in configuration of the —OH and —H on carbon atoms 2, 3 and 4 of glucose are known as

(a) Epimers (b) Anomers
(c) Optical isomers (d) Steroisomers

11. The most important epimer of glucose is

(a) Galactose (b) Fructose
(c) Arabinose (d) Xylose

12. α-D-glucose and β-D-glucose are

(a) Stereoisomers (b) Epimers
(c) Anomers (d) Keto-aldo pairs

13. α-D-glucose + 112° →+ 52.5° ←+ 19° β-D-glucose for glucose above represents

(a) Optical isomerism (b) Mutarotation
(c) Epimerisation (d) D and L isomerism

14. Compounds having the same structural formula but differing in spatial configuration are known as

(a) Stereoisomers (b) Anomers
(c) Optical isomers (d) Epimers

15. In glucose the orientation of the —H and —OH groups around the carbon atom 5 adjacent to the terminal primary alcohol carbon determines

(a) D or L series (b) Dextro or levorotatory
(c) Epimer and anomers (d) Epimers

16. The carbohydrate of the blood group substances is

(a) Sucrose (b) Fucose
(c) Arabinose (d) Maltose

17. Erythromycin contains

(a) Dimethyl amino sugar (b) Trimethyl amino sugar
(c) Sterol and sugar (d) Glycerol and sugar

18. A sugar alcohol is

(a) Mannitol (b) Trehalose
(c) Xylulose (d) Arabinose

19. The major sugar of insect hemolymph is

(a) Glycogen (b) Pectin
(c) Trehalose (d) Sucrose

20. The sugar found in DNA is

(a) Xylose (b) Ribose
(c) Deoxyribose (d) Ribulose

21. The sugar found in RNA is

(a) Ribose (b) Deoxyribose
(c) Ribulose (d) Erythrose

22. The sugar found in milk is

(a) Galactose (b) Glucose
(c) Fructose (d) Lactose

23. Invert sugar is

(a) Lactose (b) Sucrose
(c) Hydrolytic products of sucrose (d) Fructose

24. Sucrose consists of

(a) Glucose + glucose (b) Glucose + fructose
(c) Glucose + galactose (d) Glucose + mannose

25. The monosaccharide units are linked by 1 $\rightarrow$ 4 glycosidic linkage in

(a) Maltose (b) Sucrose
(c) Cellulose (d) Cellobiose

26. Which of the following is a non-reducing sugar?

(a) Isomaltose (b) Maltose
(c) Lactose (d) Trehalose

27. Which of the following is a reducing sugar?

(a) Sucrose (b) Trehalose
(c) Isomaltose (d) Agar

28. A dissaccharide formed by 1,1-glycosidic linkage between their monosaccharide units is

(a) Lactose (b) Maltose
(c) Trehalose (d) Sucrose

29. A dissaccharide formed by 1,1-glycosidic linkage between their monosaccharide units is

(a) Lactose (b) Maltose
(c) Trehalose (d) Sucrose

30. Mutarotation refers to change in

(a) pH (b) Optical rotation
(c) Conductance (d) Chemical properties

31. A polysacchharide which is often called animal starch is

(a) Glycogen (b) Starch
(c) Inulin (d) Dextrin

32. The homopolysaccharide used for intravenous infusion as plasma substitute is

(a) Agar (b) Inulin
(c) Pectin (d) Starch

33. The polysaccharide used in assessing the glomerular fittration rate (GFR) is

(a) Glycogen (b) Agar
(c) Inulin (d) Hyaluronic acid

34. The constituent unit of inulin is

(a) Glucose (b) Fructose
(c) Mannose (d) Galactose

35. The polysaccharide found in the exoskeleton of invertebrates is

(a) Pectin (b) Chitin
(c) Cellulose (d) Chondroitin sulphate

36. Which of the following is a heteroglycan?

(a) Dextrins (b) Agar
(c) Inulin (d) Chitin

37. The glycosaminoglycan which does not contain uronic acid is

(a) Dermatan sulphate (b) Chondroitin sulphate
(c) Keratan sulphate (d) Heparan sulphate

38. The glycosaminoglycan which does not contain uronic acid is

(a) Hyaluronic acid (b) Heparin
(c) Chondroitin sulphate (d) Dermatan sulphate

39. Keratan sulphate is found in abundance in

(a) Heart muscle (b) Liver
(c) Adrenal cortex (d) Cornea

40. Repeating units of hyaluronic acid are

(a) N-acetyl glucosamine and D-glucuronic acid
(b) N-acetyl galactosamine and D-glucuronic acid

(c) N-acetyl glucosamine and galactose
(d) N-acetyl galactosamine and L- iduronic acid

41. The approximate number of branches in amylopectin is

(a) 10 (b) 20
(c) 40 (d) 80

42. In amylopectin the intervals of glucose units of each branch is

(a) 10–20 (b) 24–30
(c) 30–40 (d) 40–50

43. A polymer of glucose synthesized by the action of leuconostoc mesenteroids in a sucrose medium is

(a) Dextrans (b) Dextrin
(c) Limit dextrin (d) Inulin

44. Glucose on reduction with sodium amalgam forms

(a) Dulcitol (b) Sorbitol
(c) Mannitol (d) Mannitol and sorbitol

45. Glucose on oxidation does not give

(a) Glycoside (b) Glucosaccharic acid
(c) Gluconic acid (d) Glucuronic acid

46. Oxidation of galactose with conc HNO_3 yields

(a) Mucic acid (b) Glucuronic acid
(c) Saccharic acid (d) Gluconic acid

47. A positive Benedict's test is not given by

(a) Sucrose (b) Lactose
(c) Maltose (d) Glucose

48. Starch is a

(a) Polysaccharide (b) Monosaccharide
(c) Disaccharide (d) None of these

49. A positive Seliwanoff's test is obtained with

(a) Glucose (b) Fructose
(c) Lactose (d) Maltose

50. Osazones are not formed with the

(a) Glucose (b) Fructose
(c) Sucrose (d) Lactose

Answers

1	(a)	14	(a)	27	(c)	40	(a)
2	(a)	15	(a)	28	(c)	41	(d)
3	(a)	16	(b)	29	(b)	42	(b)
4	(a)	17	(a)	30	(b)	43	(a)
5	(b)	18	(a)	31	(d)	44	(b)
6	(a)	19	(c)	32	(a)	45	(a)
7	(a)	20	(c)	33	(c)	46	(a)
8	(d)	21	(a)	34	(b)	47	(a)
9	(a)	22	(d)	35	(b)	48	(a)
10	(a)	23	(c)	36	(b)	49	(b)
11	(a)	24	(b)	37	(c)	50	(c)
12	(c)	25	(a)	38	(b)		
13	(b)	26	(d)	39	(d)		

Chapter 10
Lipids

1. **Synthesis of fatty acid takes place when**
   (a) Fatty acid are plentiful
   (b) Carbohydrate is plentiful
   (c) Carbohydrate and energy are plentiful
   (d) None of these

2. **Triacylglycerols are**
   (a) Soluble in water
   (b) Insoluble in water
   (c) Soluble in water at elevated temperature
   (d) Partially soluble in water

3. **Cholestrol is the precursor of**
   (a) Steroid hormones
   (b) Vitamin A
   (c) Bile salts
   (d) Both (a) and (c)

4. **How many classes of steroid hormones are there?**
   (a) 3
   (b) 2
   (c) 4
   (d) 5

5. **Which of the following is called milk ejection hormone?**
   (a) Prolactin
   (b) Vasopressin
   (c) Oxytocin
   (d) All of these

6. **How many types of lipoproteins are there?**
   (a) 2
   (b) 6
   (c) 8
   (d) 5

7. **HDLs are synthesized in**
   (a) Blood
   (b) Liver
   (c) Intestine
   (d) Pancreas

8. **VLDLs are synthesized in**
   (a) Blood (b) Liver
   (c) Intestine (d) Pancreas

9. **Chylomicrons are synthesized in**
   (a) Blood (b) Liver
   (c) Intestine (d) Pancreas

10. **What is the major protein constituent of high-density lipoprotein (HDL)?**
   (a) Apolipoprotein A-1 (b) Apolipoprotein C-1
   (c) Apolipoprotein E (d) None of these

11. **Atherosclerosis can cause blood**
   (a) Thinning (b) Clotting
   (c) Thickening (d) None of these

12. **Cholesterolemia means**
   (a) Lack of functional LDL receptors
   (b) Lack of functional HDL receptor
   (c) High sensitivity to fatty food intake
   (d) None of the above

13. **Arachidonate has 20 carbon atoms with**
   (a) 3 double bonds (b) 2 double bonds
   (c) 4 double bonds (d) 8 double bonds

14. **How many ATPs are formed during complete oxidation of Palmitate?**
   (a) 35 (b) 96
   (c) 129 (d) 131

15. **Fatty acid synthesis takes place in**
   (a) Mitochondria (b) Cell membrane
   (c) Cytosol (d) Endoplasmic reticulum

Answers

1	(c)	5	(c)	9	(c)	13	(c)
2	(b)	6	(d)	10	(a)	14	(c)
3	(d)	7	(a)	11	(b)	15	(c)
4	(d)	8	(b)	12	(a)		

Chapter 11

TCA Cycle

1. **Citric acid cycle occurs in**
   (a) Cytoplasm
   (b) Mitochondria
   (c) Endoplasmic reticulum
   (d) Golgi bodies
2. **How many ATPs are produced during citric acid cycle?**
   (a) 10
   (b) 13
   (c) 12
   (d) 8
3. **In what form does the product of glycolysis enter the TCA cycle?**
   (a) AcetylCoA
   (b) Pyruvate
   (c) NADH
   (d) Glucose
4. **Why the TCA cycle is the central pathway of metabolism of the cell?**
   (a) It occurs in the center of the cell
   (b) Its intermediates are commonly used by other metabolic reactions
   (c) All other metabolic pathways depend upon it
   (d) None of the above
5. **The first intermediate in TCA cycle is**
   (a) Succinate
   (b) Fumerate
   (c) Citrate
   (d) Malate
6. **In eukaryotes, electron transport occurs in**
   (a) Membranes of mitochondria
   (b) Endoplasmic reticulum
   (c) Cytoplasm
   (d) All of the above
7. **Important function of cholesterol is to**
   (a) Modulate fluidity
   (b) Enhance blood circulation
   (c) Prevent bile salts formation
   (d) None of these

8. Cholesterol can be synthesized *de novo* in

(a) Pancreas (b) Intestine

(c) Liver (d) Cell membrane

9. Oxidation of a molecule involves

(a) Gain of electron (b) Loss of electron

(c) Gain of proton (d) Loss of proton

10. A positive redox potential means substance has

(a) Lower affinity for electron (b) Higher affinity for electron

(c) Lower affinity for proton (d) Higher affinity for proton

11. Which one of the following is not the intermediate of Kreb's cycle?

(a) Isocitrate (b) Succinate

(c) Fumarate (d) Stearate

12. Which of the following enzyme does not take part in the TCA cycle?

(a) Citrate synthase (b) Iso-citrate dehydrogenase

(c) Pyruvate dehydrogenase (d) Malate dehydrogenase

13. Standard redox potential for a substance is measured under standard condition and is expressed as

(a) Mili-Ampere (b) Volt

(c) Without unit (d) Ohm

14. Which one is not the main protein in electron transport chain?

(a) NADH dehydrogenase (b) Cytochrome bcl complex

(c) Cytochrome oxidase (d) Citrate synthease

15. Given the following redox couples and standard oxidation-reduction potentials:

	E′0 (V)
2 cytochrome c ox +2 e- ←>2 cytochrome c red	**+0.254V**
2 cytochrome a.3ox + 2 e- ←>2 cytochrome a 3 red	**+0.385V**

which way would electrons move between these couples under standard conditions?

(a) From cytochrome c red to cytochrome a 3 ox

(b) From cytochrome a 3 red to cytochrome c ox

(c) From cytochrome c red to cytochrome c ox

(d) From cytochrome a 3 red to cytochrome a 3 ox

16. How many molecules ofATPs are synthesized per NADH oxidation?

(a) 2
(b) 1
(c) 3
(d) 4

17. To stop ATP synthesis which chemical is generally used?

(a) DNSA
(b) 2,4 dinitrophenol
(c) DDT
(d) None of the chemical can stop ATP synthesis

18. Malate-asparatate shuttle operates in

(a) Lungs and liver
(b) Heart and liver
(c) Pancreas and liver
(d) None of these

19. The enzymes of the TCA cycle in a eukaryotic cell are located in the

(a) Nucleus
(b) Mitochondria
(c) Plasma membrane
(d) Lysosomal bodies

20. Which of the following is involved in energy production?

(a) Generation of proton gradients across membranes
(b) Transport of electrons on organic molecules
(c) Conversion of compounds with high energy to those of low energy
(d) All of the above

21. Most multi-cellular organisms obtain energy for the synthesis ofATP during oxidative phosphorylation from

(a) High energy phosphate compounds
(b) A proton gradient across the inner mitochondrial membrane
(c) A proton gradient across the cell membrane
(d) A proton gradient across the outer mitochondrial membrane

22. The catabolism of sugars and fatty acids is similar because

(a) Both of these compounds are funnelled through the TCA/citric acid cycle
(b) Both of these compounds generate redox energy during catabolism
(c) Both of these compounds generate chemical energy during catabolism
(d) All of the above

23. Most of the enzymes of the citric acid cycle in a eukaryotic cell are located in the

(a) Inner mitochondrial membrane
(b) Cytosol
(c) Mitochondrial matrix
(d) Intermembrane space

24. **The end product of glycolysis is pyruvate, which enters the citric acid cycle after being converted to**
    (a) Acetic acid (b) Acetyl-CoA
    (c) Acetaldehyde (d) None of these

25. **During cellular respiration, most of the ATP made, is generated by**
    (a) Oxidative phosphorylation (b) Photophosphorylation
    (c) Substrate-level phosphorylation (d) Glycolysis

26. **The $FADH_2$ and NADH produced by the oxidation of one acetyl-CoA results in the synthesis of about**
    (a) 3 ATPs (b) 6 ATPs
    (c) 11 ATPs (d) 15 ATPs

27. **Energy that is released from glucose during respiration but not transferred to ATP bonds can be detected as**
    (a) CO_2 (b) AMP
    (c) ADP (d) Heat

Answers

1	(b)	8	(c)	15	(a)	22	(a)
2	(c)	9	(b)	16	(c)	23	(c)
3	(a)	10	(b)	17	(b)	24	(b)
4	(b)	11	(d)	18	(b)	25	(a)
5	(c)	12	(c)	19	(b)	26	(c)
6	(a)	13	(b)	20	(d)	27	(d)
7	(b)	14	(d)	21	(b)		

Chapter 12
Protein and Protein Metabolism

1. **All proteins contain the**
   (a) Same 20 amino acids
   (b) Different amino acids
   (c) 300 Amino acids occurring in nature
   (d) Only a few amino acids

2. **Proteins contain**
   (a) Only L-amino acids
   (b) Only D-amino acids
   (c) DL-Amino acids
   (d) Both (a) and (b)

3. **The optically inactive amino acid is**
   (a) Glycine
   (b) Serine
   (c) Threonine
   (d) Valine

4. **At neutral pH, a mixture of amino acids in solution would be predominantly**
   (a) Dipolar ions
   (b) Nonpolar molecules
   (c) Positive and monovalent
   (d) Hydrophobic

5. **The true statement about solutions of amino acids at physiological pH is**
   (a) All amino acids contain both positive and negative charges
   (b) All amino acids contain positively charged side chains
   (c) Some amino acids contain only positive charge
   (d) All amino acids contain negatively charged side chains

6. **pH (isoelectric pH) of alanine is**
   (a) 6.02
   (b) 6.6
   (c) 6.8
   (d) 7.2

7. **Since the pK values for aspartic acid are 2.0, 3.9 and 10.0, it follows that the isoelectric (pH) is**
   (a) 3.0
   (b) 3.9
   (c) 5.9
   (d) 6.0

8. **Sulphur containing amino acid is**
   (a) Methionine (b) Leucine
   (c) Valine (d) Asparagine

9. **An example of sulphur containing amino acid is**
   (a) 2-Amino-3-mercaptopropanoic acid
   (b) 2-Amino-3-methylbutanoic acid
   (c) 2-Amino-3-hydroxypropanoic acid
   (d) Amino acetic acid

10. **All the following are sulphur containing amino acids found in proteins except**
   (a) Cysteine (b) Cystine
   (c) Methionine (d) Threonine

11. **An aromatic amino acid is**
   (a) Lysine (b) Tyrosine
   (c) Taurine (d) Arginine

12. **The functions of plasma albumin are**
   (a) Osmosis (b) Transport
   (c) Immunity (d) Both (a) and (b)

13. **Amino acid with side chain containing basic groups is**
   (a) 2-Amino 5-guanidovaleric acid
   (b) 2-Pyrrolidine carboxylic acid
   (c) 2-Amino 3-mercaptopropanoic acid
   (d) 2-Amino propanoic acid

14. **An example of L-amino acid not present in proteins but essential in mammalian metabolism is**
   (a) 3-Amino 3-hydroxypropanoic acid
   (b) 2-Amino 3-hydroxybutanoic acid
   (c) 2-Amino 4-mercaptobutanoic acid
   (d) 2-Amino 3-mercaptopropanoic acid

15. **An essential amino acid in man is**
   (a) Aspartate (b) Tyrosine
   (c) Methionine (d) Serine

16. **Non essential amino acids**
   (a) Are not components of tissue proteins
   (b) May be synthesized in the body from essential amino acids

(c) Have no role in the metabolism
(d) May be synthesized in the body in diseased states

17. Which one of the following is semiessential amino acid for humans?
(a) Valine (b) Arginine
(c) Lysine (d) Tyrosine

18. An example of polar amino acid is
(a) Alanine (b) Leucine
(c) Arginine (d) Valine

19. The amino acid with a nonpolar side chain is
(a) Serine (b) Valine
(c) Asparagine (d) Threonine

20. A ketogenic amino acid is
(a) Valine (b) Cysteine
(c) Leucine (d) Threonine

21. An amino acid that does not form an α-helix is
(a) Valine (b) Proline
(c) Tyrosine (d) Tryptophan

22. An amino acid not found in proteins is
(a) L-Alanine (b) Proline
(c) Lysine (d) Histidine

23. In mammalian tissues serine can be a biosynthetic precursor of
(a) Methionine (b) Glycine
(c) Tryptophan (d) Phenylalanine

24. A vasodilating compound is produced by the decarboxylation of the amino acid
(a) Arginine (b) Aspartic acid
(c) Glutamine (d) Histidine

25. Biuret reaction is specific for
(a) –CONH-linkages (b) $-CSNH_2$ group
(c) $-(NH)NH_2$ group (d) All of these

26. Sakaguchi's reaction is specific for
(a) Tyrosine (b) Proline
(c) Arginine (d) Cysteine

27. Million-Nasse's reaction is specific for the amino acid
(a) Tryptophan (b) Tyrosine
(c) Phenylalanine (d) Arginine

28. Ninhydrin with evolution of CO_2 forms a blue complex with
(a) Peptide bond (b) L-Amino acids
(c) Serotonin (d) Histamine

29. The most of the ultraviolet absorption of proteins above 240 nm is due to their content of
(a) Tryptophan (b) Aspartate
(c) Glutamate (d) Alanine

30. Which of the following is a dipeptide?
(a) Anserine (b) Glutathione
(c) Glucagon (d) L-Lipoprotein

31. Which of the following is a tripeptide?
(a) Anserine (b) Oxytocin
(c) Glutathione (d) Kallidin

32. A peptide which acts as potent smooth muscle hypotensive agent is
(a) Glutathione (b) Bradykinin
(c) Tryocidine (d) Gramicidin-s

33. A tripeptide functioning as an important reducing agent in the tissues is
(a) Bradykinin (b) Kallidin
(c) Tyrocidin (d) Glutathione

34. An example of metalloprotein is
(a) Casein (b) Ceruloplasmin
(c) Gelatin (d) Salmine

35. Carbonic anhydrase is an example of
(a) Lipoprotein (b) Phosphoprotein
(c) Metalloprotein (d) Chromoprotein

36. An example of chromoprotein is
(a) Haemoglobin (b) Sturine
(c) Nuclein (d) Gliadin

37. An example of scleroprotein is
(a) Zein (b) Keratin
(c) Glutenin (d) Ovoglobulin

38. Casein, the milk protein is

(a) Nucleoprotein (b) Chromoprotein

(c) Phosphoprotein (d) Glycoprotein

39. An example of phosphoprotein presen in egg yolk is

(a) Ovoalbumin (b) Ovoglobulin

(c) Ovovitellin (d) Avidin

40. A simple protein found in the nucleoproteins of the sperm is

(a) Prolamine (b) Protamine

(c) Glutelin (d) Globulin

41. Histones are

(a) Identical to protamine

(b) Proteins rich in lysine and arginine

(c) Proteins with high molecular weight

(d) Insoluble in water and very dilute acids

42. The protein present in hair is

(a) Keratin (b) Elastin

(c) Myosin (d) Tropocollagen

43. The amino acid from which synthesis of the protein of hair keratin takes place is

(a) Alanine (b) Methionine

(c) Proline (d) Hydroxyproline

44. In one molecule of albumin the number of amino acids is

(a) 510 (b) 590

(c) 610 (d) 650

45. Plasma proteins which contain more than 4 per cent hexosamine are

(a) Microglobulins (b) Glycoproteins

(c) Mucoproteins (d) Orosomucoids

46. After releasing O_2 at the tissues, hemoglobin transports

(a) CO_2 and protons to the lungs (b) O_2 to the lungs

(c) CO_2 and protons to the tissue (d) Nutrients

47. Ehlers-Danlos syndrome characterized by hypermobile joints and skin abnormalities is due to

(a) Abnormality in gene for procollagen

(b) Deficiency of lysyl oxidase

(c) Deficiency of prolyl hydroxylase
(d) Deficiency of lysyl hydroxylase

48. Proteins are soluble in

(a) Anhydrous acetone
(b) Aqueous alcohol
(c) Anhydrous alcohol
(d) Benzene

49. A cereal protein soluble in 70 per cent alcohol but insoluble in water or salt solution is

(a) Glutelin
(b) Protamine
(c) Albumin
(d) Gliadin

50. Many globular proteins are stable in solution inspite they lack in

(a) Disulphide bonds
(b) Hydrogen bonds
(c) Salt bonds
(d) Non polar bonds

Answers

1	(a)	14	(c)	27	(b)	40	(b)
2	(a)	15	(c)	28	(b)	41	(b)
3	(a)	16	(b)	29	(a)	42	(a)
4	(a)	17	(b)	30	(a)	43	(b)
5	(a)	18	(c)	31	(c)	44	(c)
6	(a)	19	(b)	32	(b)	45	(c)
7	(a)	20	(c)	33	(d)	46	(a)
8	(a)	21	(b)	34	(b)	47	(a)
9	(a)	22	(a)	35	(c)	48	(b)
10	(d)	23	(b)	36	(a)	49	(d)
11	(b)	24	(d)	37	(b)	50	(a)
12	(a)	25	(a)	38	(c)		
13	(a)	26	(c)	39	(c)		

Chapter 13
Protein Structure

1. **Beta pleated sheets are examples of protein's**
   (a) Primary structure
   (b) Secondary structure
   (c) Tertiary structure
   (d) Quaternary structure

2. **The four subunits of the haemoglobin (Hb) gene represent protein's**
   (a) Primary structure
   (b) Secondary structure
   (c) Tertiary structure
   (d) Quaternary structure

3. **Protein folding is**
   (a) Automatic, mediated by the protein itself
   (b) Mediated by other proteins called chaperones
   (c) Mediated by the ribosomes
   (d) None of the above

4. **Signal sequences are part of a protcin that**
   (a) Signal folding of the protein
   (b) Signal the protein synthesis on the ribosomes is ended
   (c) Transport proteins to other sites within the cell
   (d) Refold proteins in prion-associated diseases

5. **Individuals with PKU disease are mentally retarded unless**
   (a) Phenylalanine in the diet is restricted
   (b) Tyrosine in the diet is restricted
   (c) Homogentisic acid in the diet is restricted
   (d) None of the above

6. **Sickle cell disease is due to**
   (a) A mutation in the beta chain of Hb
   (b) Infection with a parasite
   (c) A mutation in the alpha chain of Hb
   (d) None of the above

7. **Marfan's syndrome is thought to be a mutation affecting**
   (a) Haemoglobin synthesis
   (b) Collagen synthesis
   (c) Metabolism of homogentisic acid
   (d) Insufficient thyroid production

8. **Over 50 per cent of common cancers are associated with damage to a protein, p53. This protein**
   (a) Is a cyclin
   (b) Is a tumor supressor
   (c) Is an oncogene
   (d) Regulates apoptosis

9. **Cyclins are proteins that**
   (a) Regulate ability of cells to invade tissue
   (b) Regulate passage from one stage of cell division to another
   (c) Regulate apoptosis of damaged cells
   (d) None of the above

10. **BRACI, an inherited form of breast cancer, regulates cell division by**
   (a) Binding to a DNA sequence
   (b) Complexing with cyclins
   (c) Binding to the cell outer membrane
   (d) Binding to the protein RAD 51 which repairs DNA damage

11. **Metastasis involves**
   (a) Ability of cells to dissolve cellular matrix
   (b) Metalloprotein levels
   (c) Decreased levels of proteins that regulate metalloproteins
   (d) All of the above

12. **Different DNA polymerases play distinct roles in DNA replication and repair in both prokaryotic and eukaryotic cells. All known DNA polymerases synthesize DNA only in the by the addition of dNTPs to a performed primer strand of DNA.**
   (a) Positive direction
   (b) 3' to 5' direction
   (c) 5' to 3' direction
   (d) Negative direction

13. **Reverse transcriptase from HIV does not**
   (a) Uses RNA as a template
   (b) Has a 5' to 3' polymerase activity
   (c) Has a 3'- 5' exonuclease activity
   (d) Requires a primer

14. Which of the following amino acids interact with the DNA or RNA backbone (*i.e.* phosphate)?

(a) Ile and Val (b) Lys and Arg
(c) Leu and Ala (d) Cys and Met

15. Which of the following amino acids can interact with the DNA or RNA nucleotide bases via hydrogen bonding?

(a) Asn and Gln (b) Cys and Met
(c) Lys and Leu (d) Ile and Val

16. The type II restriction endonucleases, bind to DNA sites

(a) Using H-bonds for specificity
(b) That are usually palindromic
(c) Using non-sequence-dependent backbone interactions
(d) All of the above

17. Cleavage of DNA by EcoRl endonuclease results in the formation of

(a) Two 3'-OH ends and two 5'-phosphate ends
(b) One 3'-OH end and one 5'-phosphate end
(c) Two 3'-phosphate ends and two 3'-OH ends
(d) One 3'-OH end and two 5'-phosphate end

18. The enzyme that joins DNA cuts is called

(a) Joinase (b) Ligase
(c) DNA phosphorylase (d) Reverse transcriptase

Answers

1	(b)	6	(a)	11	(d)	16	(d)
2	(d)	7	(b)	12	(c)	17	(a)
3	(b)	8	(b)	13	(c)	18	(b)
4	(c)	9	(b)	14	(b)		
5	(a)	10	(d)	15	(a)		

Chapter 14
Nitrogen Metabolism

1. **How many molecules of ATP are hydrolysed to form two molecule of ammonia?**
   (a) 10 (b) 5
   (c) 16 (d) 15

2.Nitrate reduction can be carried out by
   (a) Only microorganism (b) Plant and microorganism
   (c) Only plants (d) None of these

3. **Which of the following amino acid do not fall under the category of essential amino acid?**
   (a) Histidine (b) Leucine
   (c) Glycine (d) Methionine

4. **The inputs to one cycle of the urea cycle are**
   (a) 1 molecule of aspartic acid, 1 molecule of ammonia, 1 molecule of carbon dioxide, 3 molecules of ATP
   (b) 1 molecule of urea, l molecule of ammonia, 3 molecules of ATP and 1 molecule of fumaric acid
   (c) 1 molecule of fumaric acid, 1 molecule of urea, 3 molecules of AMP
   (d) None of the above

5. **The products of urea cycle are**
   (a) 1 molecule of urea, 1 molecule of ammonia, 1 molecule of ATP and 1 molecule of fumaric acid
   (b) 1 molecule of fumaric acid, 1 molecule of urea, 1 molecule of AMP, 2 molecules of ADP
   (c) 1 molecule ofaspartic acid, 1 molecule of ammonia, 1 molecule of fumaric acid, 1 molecule of ATP
   (d) None of the above

6. **Urea cycle converts**
   (a) Ammonia into a less toxic form (b) Ketoacids into amino acids
   (c) Amino acids into ketoacids (d) None of these
7. **The nitrogen atoms of urea produced in the urea cycle are derived from**
   (a) Nitrate (b) Ammonia and aspartic acid
   (c) Nitrite (d) Ammonia
8. **Which of the following is used as carbon atom source while producing urea in the urea cycle?**
   (a) Arginine (b) Aspartic acid
   (c) Carbon dioxide (d) Glucose
9. **Transaminase enzymes are present in**
   (a) Liver (b) Pancreas
   (c) Intestine (d) None of these
10. **Key enzyme of N_2 metabolism is**
    (a) Nitrate reductase (b) Nitrite reductase
    (c) Glutamate synthase (d) None of these
11. **A best described ketogenic amino acid is**
    (a) Lysine (b) Tryptophan
    (c) Valine (d) None of these
12. **The most toxic compounds is**
    (a) Tyrosine (b) Phenylpyruvate
    (c) Lysine (d) Phenylalanine
13. **In the normal breakdown of Pennylalanine, it is initially degraded to**
    (a) Fumarate (b) Tyrosine
    (c) Lysine (d) Phenylpyruvate
14. **Which of the following amino acids is considered as both ketogenic and glucogenic?**
    (a) Vapine (b) Tryptophan
    (c) Lysine (d) None of these

Answers

1	(c)	5	(b)	9	(a)	13	(b)
2	(b)	6	(a)	10	(a)	14	(b)
3	(c)	7	(b)	11	(a)		
4	(a)	8	(c)	12	(b)		

Chapter 15
Nitrogen Fixation and Photosynthesis

1. **The chief source of nitrogen for green plants is**
   (a) Atmospheric nitrogen
   (b) Nitrates
   (c) Ammonium salts
   (d) Low molecular weight- organic nitrogenous compound

2. **In the presence of carbon monoxide, nitrogen fixation**
   (a) Increases (b) Decreases
   (c) Inhibits (d) None of these

3. **Plants absorb nitrates from soil and convert them into**
   (a) Urea (b) Ammonia
   (c) Nitrogen (d) None of these

4. **Nitrosomonous and Nitrobacter obtain their carbon for growth from**
   (a) Organic compounds (b) Carbon dioxide
   (c) Elementary carbon (d) None of these

5. **Which of the following aid plants in the acquisition of nitrogen from nitrogen gas of the atmosphere?**
   (a) Bacteria (b) Algae
   (c) Nematodes (d) Moulds

6. **During nitrogen fixation the enzyme nitrogenase catalyse the reaction. The reaction is high energy demanding which require approximately**
   (a) 12 ATP (b) 18ATP
   (c) 25ATP (d) 7ATP

7. **A major plant macronutrient found in nucleic acids and proteins is**
   (a) Calcium (b) Nitrogen
   (c) Sulphur (d) Iron

8. **Organisms capable of converting N_2 to NO_3 are**
   (a) Yeasts (b) Bacteria
   (c) Roundworms (d) Moulds

9. **Which of the following bacteria genus is capable of oxidizing ammonia (NH_4)?**
   (a) Nitrospina (b) Nitrobacter
   (c) Nitrosococcus (d) Nitrosobacter

10. **Which of the following molecule is produced from the fixation of CO_2 in C_4 plants?**
    (a) Malate (b) Oxal
    (c) Pyruvate (d) Alpha-ketoglutarate

11. **The following are the products of the light reactions of photosynthesis except**
    (a) ATP (b) Oxygen
    (c) NADPH (d) Glucose

12. **$NADP^+$ is recued to NADPH during**
    (a) Light dependent reactions (b) Photorespiration
    (c) Calvin cycle (d) None of these

13. **Carbon dioxide is reduced in**
    (a) Noncyclic photophosphorylation (b) The calvin cycle
    (c) The light reactions (d) Both light and dark reaction

14. **The cytochrome C oxidase complex**
    (a) Accept electrons from cyt. C (b) Donates four electrons to O_2
    (c) Pumps protons out of the matrix space (d) All of these

15. **Hydrogen (electron) acceptor in the light reactions is**
    (a) ADP (b) $NADP^+$
    (c) NAD^+ (d) FADH

Answers

1	(b)	5	(a)	9	(c)	13	(b)
2	(c)	6	(b)	10	(b)	14	(d)
3	(b)	7	(b)	11	(d)	15	(b)
4	(b)	8	(b)	12	(a)		

Chapter 16
Vitamins and Coenzymes

1. **Vitamins are essential because the organism**
   (a) Can't synthesize these compounds at all
   (b) Can synthesize these compounds partially
   (c) Can't synthesize these compounds in the adequate amounts
   (d) None of the above

2. **The vitamin riboflavin, which occurs as a yellow pigment in egg yolk and milk become**
   (a) Colorless on reduction with Zn in acid and regained its color on re-oxidation
   (b) Colorless on oxidation and regained its color on reduction with Zn in acid
   (c) More deep in color on reduction with Zn in acid and regained its color on re-oxidation
   (d) More deep in color on oxidation and regained its color on reduction with Zn in acid

3. **A deficiency of niacin causes**
   (a) Pellagra
   (b) Scurvy
   (c) Cataract
   (d) Anemia

4. **Which of these is a symptom of vitamin A deficiency?**
   (a) Osteoporosis
   (b) Impaired taste perception
   (c) Blindness
   (d) Impaired blood clotting

5. **Which of these is a vitamin A precursor?**
   (a) Cobalamin
   (b) Pyridoxine
   (c) Beta-Carotene
   (d) Thiamine

6. **The vitamin riboflavin part of the __________ molecule.**
   (a) Ferredoxin
   (b) FAD
   (c) Pyridoxal phosphate
   (d) Pyrophosphate

7. **Vitamin niacin is part of the __________ molecule.**
   (a) Ferredoxin (b) Pyridoxal phosphate
   (c) Pyrophosphate (d) NAD

8. **Main function of insulin hormone is to**
   (a) Increase glycogen in liver (b) Decrease glycogen in
   (c) Increase blood sugar (d) Decrease blood sugar

9. **An example of a digestive hormone is**
   (a) Lipase (b) Pepsin
   (c) Amylase (d) Gastrin

10. **Which of these hormones is a catecholamine?**
    (a) Follitropin (b) Norepinephrine
    (c) Tetraiodothyronine (d) Tetrahydrofolate

11. **Which of these molecules is vitamin H?**
    (a) Biotin (b) Carnitine
    (c) Folic acid (d) None of these

12. **The occurrence of metals such as iron or molybdenum in some flavoproteins can**
    (a) Stabilize the semiquinone (b) De-stabilize the semiquinone
    (c) Form chelation (d) All of these

13. **In one iron-metalloflavoprotein, the iron is present as a**
    (a) Heme-protein (b) Non heme type
    (c) Both (a) and (b) (d) Flavin moiety

14. **Dihydroorotate dehydrogenase contains**
    (a) 4 flavins and 4 atoms of iron per molecule
    (b) 2 flavins and 4 atoms of iron per molecule
    (c) 2 flavins and 2 atoms of iron per molecule
    (d) 4 flavins and 2 atoms of iron per molecule

15. **Lipoic acid exists in**
    (a) Oxidized form (b) Reduced form
    (c) Oxidized and reduced form both (d) None of these

16. **Lipoic acid is a co-factor of the**
    (a) A-ketoglutaric dehydrogenase (b) Pyruvic dehydrogenase
    (c) Di-hydroorotate dehydrogenase (d) Both (a) and (b)

17. Biotin occurs mainly in combined forms bound to protein through

(a) E-N-lysine moiety
(b) E-S-lysine moiety
(c) S-N-biotinyl-L-lysine
(d) C-N-lipoyl - L-lysine

18. A deficiency of thiamin produces the disease known as

(a) Beri-beri
(b) Scurvy
(c) Cataract
(d) Anemia

19. Which of the following compounds/(s) belong/(s) to the vitamin B6 group?

(a) Pyridoxal
(b) Pyridoxine
(c) Pyridoxamine
(d) All of these

20. An enzyme, L-folate reductase reduces folk acid to

(a) Hydrofolic acid
(b) Dihydrofolic acid
(c) Trihydrofolic acid
(d) Tetrahydrofolic acid

21. Which of the following are reduced coenzymes?

(a) NADII and FADH2
(b) NAD^+ and FAD
(c) ATP and GTP
(d) Coenzyme A and ubiquinone

22. In the co-enzyme B_{12} the position occupied by a cyanide ion in vitamin B_{12} is bonded directly to the __________ of the ribose of adenosine.

(a) Adenine
(b) 5-6 dimethylbenzimidazole
(c) Hydroxycobalamin
(d) Cyanocobalamin

23. Vitamin B_{12} is useful in the prevention and treatment of

(a) Pernicious anemia
(b) Scurvy
(c) Cataract
(d) Beri-beri

24. The reductant, NADH, transfers the electrons via a flavo-proteins to the specific disulfide (S-S) protein to form a dithiol (SH,SH) protein which converts vitamin

(a) $B_{12}(Co^{2+})$ to $B_{12}(Co)$
(b) $B_{12}(Co)$ to $B_{12}(Co^{2+})$
(c) $B_{12}(Co^{2+})$ to $B_{12}(Co^{+})$
(d) $B_{12}(Co^{+})$ to $B_{12}(Co^{2+})$

25. Acyl carrier protein (ACP) plays an important role in the biosynthesis of

(a) Fatty acids
(b) Amino acids
(c) Sugars
(d) Carbohydrates

26. *E. coli* ACP has its molecular weight as around

(a) 9000
(b) 19000
(c) 39000
(d) 90000

27. Vitamin-C is considered as a

(a) Water soluble
(b) Fat soluble
(c) Fat and water soluble
(d) None of these

28. Who discovered vitamin C (ascorbic acid)?

(a) Paul Berg
(b) Linus Pauling
(c) Albert Szent-Gyorgyi
(d) Kerry Mullis

29. The absence of ascorbic acid in the human diet gives rise to

(a) Rickets
(b) Pernicious anemia
(c) Cataract
(d) Beri-beri

30. Ascorbic acid acts as an

(a) Reducing agent
(b) Oxidizing agent
(c) Oxidizing and reducing agent both
(d) None of the above

31. β-carotene together with α-carotene, γ-carotene and cryptoxanthine are synthesized by

(a) Plants
(b) Animal
(c) Plants and animals both
(c) None of these

32. An early sign of retinol deficiencies in man is

(a) Night blindness
(b) Keratinization
(c) Xeropthalmia
(d) None of these

33. The symptoms of retinol excess are

(a) Bone fragility
(b) Nausea
(c) Weakness
(d) All of these

34. Vitamin-D deficiency can cause

(a) Rickets
(b) Pernicious anemia
(c) Cataract
(d) Beri-beri

35. The most prominent role that tocopherol has in *in-vitro* systems is as a strong

(a) Antioxidants
(b) Reducing agent
(c) Oxidizing agent
(d) All of these

36. Selenium is an essential component of the enzyme glutathione peroxidase which

(a) Scavenges toxic hydoperoxycompounds in tissues
(b) Reduces toxic hydoperoxycompounds in tissues
(c) Oxidizes toxic hydoperoxycompounds in tissues
(d) None of the above

37. Vitamin K_1 was first isolated from alfalalfa and has the phytyl side chain consisting of

(a) Four isoprene units
(b) Six isoprene units
(c) Nine isoprene units
(d) Four isoprene units

38. A deficiency of Vitamin K results in a decreased level of

(a) Prothrombin
(b) Thrombin
(c) Fibrin
(d) Fibrinogen

39. Models of end-linked Osaka VI Fibrinogen dimers, a bilayer dimer is linked at

(a) Both ends by one disulfide bond
(b) Either end via two disulfide bonds
(c) Either end via a single disulfide bond
(d) Both ends by two disulfide bonds

40. The disease Beriberi is due to a dietary deficiency in

(a) Vitamin B_1 (thiamine)
(b) Vitamin B_2 (riboflavin)
(c) Vitamin B_6 (pyridoxine)
(d) Vitamin B_{12}

41. What metal ion is specifically bound by vitamin B12?

(a) Cobalt
(b) Copper
(c) Zinc
(d) Iron

42. What compound of raw egg white causes a syndrome similar to vitamin B deficiency?

(a) Avidin
(b) Betabindin
(c) Ovalbumin
(d) Albumin

43. Vitamin B_{12} (Cobalamin) is only synthesized by

(a) Fishes
(b) Micro-organisms
(c) Plants
(d) Animals

44. The prosthetic group biotin is a carrier of which type of molecule?

(a) Activated carbon dioxide (CO_2)
(b) Ammonia
(c) Methyl group
(d) Sulfhydryl group

45. A fat-soluble vitamin that regulates blood clotting is

(a) Vitamin A
(b) Vitamin K
(c) Vitamin C
(d) Niacin

46. What transports copper from the intestinal cells to the liver?

(a) Ceruloplasmin
(b) Secretin
(c) Acrolein
(d) Albumin

47. What condition is caused by iodine deficiency during pregnancy and is characterized by stunted growth, deafness, and mental retardation?

(a) Cretinism
(b) Keshan disease
(c) Multiple sclerosis
(d) Crohn's disease

Answers

1	(a)	13	(a)	25	(a)	37	(a)
2	(a)	14	(a)	26	(a)	38	(a)
3	(a)	15	(c)	27	(a)	39	(d)
4	(c)	16	(c)	28	(c)	40	(a)
5	(c)	17	(a)	29	(b)	41	(a)
6	(b)	18	(a)	30	(a)	42	(a)
7	(d)	19	(d)	31	(a)	43	(b)
8	(d)	20	(b)	32	(a)	44	(a)
9	(d)	21	(a)	33	(d)	45	(b)
10	(b)	22	(a)	34	(a)	46	(a)
11	(a)	23	(a)	35	(a)	47	(a)
12	(a)	24	(c)	36	(a)		

Chapter 17
Vitamins

1. **Vitamins are**
   (a) Accessory food factors
   (b) Generally synthesized in the body
   (c) Produced in endocrine glands
   (d) Proteins in nature

2. **Vitamin A or retinal is a**
   (a) Steroid
   (b) Polyisoprenoid compound containing a cyclohexenyl ring
   (c) Benzoquinone derivative
   (d) 6-Hydroxychromane

3. **β-Carotene, precursor of vitamin A, is oxidatively cleaved by**
   (a) β-Carotene dioxygenase (b) Oxygenase
   (c) Hydroxylase (d) Transferase

4. **Retinal is reduced to retinol in intestinal mucosa by a specific retinaldehyde reductase utilising**
   (a) $NADPH + H^+$ (b) FAD
   (c) NAD (d) $NADH + H^+$

5. **Preformed Vitamin A is supplied by**
   (a) Milk, fat and liver (b) All yellow vegetables
   (c) All yellow fruits (d) Leafy green vegetables

6. **Retinol and retinal are interconverted requiring dehydrogenase or reductase in the presence of**
   (a) NAD or NADP (b) NADH + H+
   (c) NADPH (d) FAD

7. **Fat soluble vitamins are**
   (a) Soluble in alcohol
   (b) One or more Propene units
   (c) Stored in liver
   (d) All these

8. **The international unit of vitamin A is equivalent to the activity caused by**
   (a) 0.3 μg of Vitamin A alcohol
   (b) 0.344 μg of Vitamin A alcohol
   (c) 0.6 μg of Vitamin A alcohol
   (d) 1.0 μg of Vitamin A alcohol

9. **Lumirhodopsin is stable only at temperature below**
   (a) –10°C
   (b) –20°C
   (c) –40°C
   (d) –50°C

10. **Retinol is transported in blood bound to**
    (a) Aporetinol binding protein
    (b) α-Globulin
    (c) γ-Globulin
    (d) Albumin

11. **The normal serum concentration of vitamin A in mg/100 ml is**
    (a) 5–10
    (b) 15–60
    (c) 100–150
    (d) 0–5

12. **One manifestation of vitamin A deficiency is**
    (a) Painful joints
    (b) Night blindness
    (c) Loss of hair
    (d) Thickening of long bones

13. **Deficiency of Vitamin A causes**
    (a) Xeropthalmia
    (b) Hypoprothrombinemia
    (c) Megaloblastic anemia
    (d) Pernicious anemia

14. **An important function of vitamin A is**
    (a) To act as coenzyme for a few enzymes
    (b) To play an integral role in protein synthesis
    (c) To prevent haemorrhages
    (d) To maintain the integrity of epithelial tissue

15. **Retinal is a component of**
    (a) Iodopsin
    (b) Rhodopsin
    (c) Cardiolipin
    (d) Glycoproteins

16. **Retinoic acid participates in the synthesis of**
    (a) Iodopsin
    (b) Rhodopsin
    (c) Glycoprotein
    (d) Cardiolipin

17. On exposure to light rhodopsin forms
(a) All trans-retinal
(b) Cis-retinal
(c) Retinol
(d) Retinoic acid

18. Carr-Price reaction is used to detect
(a) Vitamin A
(b) Vitamin D
(c) Ascorbic acid
(d) Vitamin E

19. The structure shown below is of
(a) Cholecalciferol
(b) 25-Hydroxycholecalciferol
(c) Ergocalciferol
(d) 7-Dehydrocholesterol

20. Vitamin D absorption is increased in
(a) Acid pH of intestine
(b) Alkaline pH of intestine
(c) Impaired fat absorption
(d) Contents of diet

21. The most potent Vitamin D metabolite is
(a) 25-Hydroxycholecalciferol
(b) 1,25-Dihydroxycholecalciferol
(c) 24, 25-Dihydroxycholecalciferol
(d) 7-Dehydrocholesterol

22. The normal serum concentration of 25-hydroxycholecalciferol in ng/ml is
(a) 0–8
(b) 60–100
(c) 100–150
(d) 8–55

23. The normal serum concentration of 1,25-dihydroxycholecalciferol in pg/ml is
(a) 26–65
(b) 1–5
(c) 5–20
(d) 80–100

24. The normal serum concentration of 24,25-dihydroxycholecalciferol in ng/ml is
(a) 8–20
(b) 25–50
(c) 1–5
(d) 60–100

25. A poor source of Vitamin D is
(a) Egg
(b) Butter
(c) Milk
(d) Liver

26. Richest source of Vitamin D is
(a) Fish liver oils
(b) Margarine
(c) Egg yolk
(d) Butter

27. Deficiency of vitamin D causes

(a) Ricket and osteomalacia
(b) Tuberculosis of bone
(c) Hypthyroidism
(d) Skin cancer

28. One international unit (I.U.) of vitamin D is defined as the biological activity of

(a) 0.025 μg of cholecalciferol
(b) 0.025 μg of 7-dehydrocholecalciferol
(c) 0.025 μg of ergosterol
(d) 0.025 μg of ergocalciferol

29. The L-ring of 7-dehydrocholesterol is cleaved to form cholecalciferol by

(a) Infrared light
(b) Dim light
(c) Ultraviolet irridation with sunlight
(d) Light of the tube lights

30. Calcitriol synthesis involves

(a) Both liver and kidney
(b) Intestine
(c) Adipose tissue
(d) Muscle

31. Insignificant amount of Vitamin E is present in

(a) Wheat germ oil
(b) Sunflower seed oil
(c) Safflower seed oil
(d) Fish liver oil

32. The activity of tocopherols is destroyed by

(a) Commercial cooking
(b) Reduction
(c) Conjugation
(d) All of these

33. The requirement of Vitamin E is increased with greater intake of

(a) Carbohydrates
(b) Proteins
(c) Polyunsaturated fat
(d) Saturated fat

34. Vitamin E reduces the requirement of

(a) Iron
(b) Zinc
(c) Selenium
(d) Magnesium

35. The most important natural antioxidant is

(a) Vitamin D
(b) Vitamin E
(c) Vitamin B_{12}
(d) Vitamin K

36. Tocopherols prevent the oxidation of

(a) Vitamin A
(b) Vitamin D
(c) Vitamin K
(d) Vitamin C

37. Creatinuria is caused due to the deficiency of vitamin

(a) A (b) K

(c) E (d) D

38. All the following conditions produce a real or functional deficiency of vitamin K except

(a) Prolonged oral, broad spectrum antibiotic therapy

(b) Total lack of red meat in the diet

(c) The total lack of green leafy vegetables in the diet

(d) Being a new born infant

39. Vitamin K is found in

(a) Green leafy plants (b) Meat

(c) Fish (d) Milk

40. Function of Vitamin A

(a) Healing epithelial tissues (b) Protein synthesis regulation

(c) Cell growth (d) All of these

41. Vitamin K_2 was originally isolated from

(a) Soyabean (b) Wheat gram

(c) Alfa Alfa (d) Putrid fish meal

42. Vitamin synthesized by bacterial in the intestine is

(a) A (b) C

(c) D (d) K

43. Vitamin K is involved in posttranslational modification of the blood clotting factors by acting as cofactor for the enzyme

(a) Carboxylase (b) Decarboxylase

(c) Hydroxylase (d) Oxidase

44. Vitamin K is a cofactor for

(a) Gamma carboxylation of glutamic acid residue

(b) β-oxidation of fatty acid

(c) Formation of ?-amino butyrate

(d) Synthesis of tryptophan

45. Hypervitaminosis K in neonates may cause

(a) Porphyria (b) Jaundice

(c) Pellagra (d) Prolonged bleeding

46. Dicoumarol is antagonist to

(a) Riboflavin (b) Retinol

(c) Menadione (d) Tocopherol

47. In the individuals who are given liberal quantities of vitamin C, the serum ascorbic acid level is

(a) 1–1.4 μg/100 ml (b) 2–4 μg/100 ml

(c) 1–10 μg/100 ml (d) 10–20 μg/100 ml

48. The vitamin which would most likely become deficient in an individual who develop a completely carnivorous life style is

(a) Thiamin (b) Niacin

(c) Vitamin C (d) Cobalamin

49. In human body highest concentration of ascorbic acid is found in

(a) Liver (b) Adrenal cortex

(c) Adrenal medulla (d) Spleen

50. The vitamin required for the formation of hydroxyproline (in collagen) is

(a) Vitamin C (b) Vitamin A

(c) Vitamin D (d) Vitamin E

51. Vitamin required for the conversion of p-hydroxyphenylpyruvate to homogentisate is

(a) Folacin (b) Cobalamin

(c) Ascorbic acid (d) Niacin

52. Vitamin required in conversion of folic acid to folinic acid is

(a) Biotin (b) Cobalamin

(c) Ascorbic acid (d) Niacin

53. Ascorbic acid can reduce

(a) 2, 6-Dibromobenzene (b) 2, 6-Diiodoxypyridine

(c) 2, 6-Dichlorophenol indophenol (d) 2, 4-Dinitrobenzene

54. Sterilised milk lacks in

(a) Vitamin A (b) Vitamin D

(c) Vitamin C (d) Thiamin

55. Scurvy is caused due to the deficiency of

(a) Vitamin A (b) Vitamin D

(c) Vitamin K (d) Vitamin C

56. Both Wernicke's disease and beriberi can be reversed by administrating

(a) Retinol (b) Thiamin

(c) Pyridoxine (d) Vitamin B_{12}

57. The Vitamin B_1 deficiency causes

(a) Ricket (b) Nyctalopia

(c) Beriberi (d) Pellagra

58. Concentration of pyruvic acid and lactic acid in blood is increased due to deficiency of the vitamin

(a) Thiamin (b) Riboflavin

(c) Niacin (d) Pantothenic acid

59. Vitamin B_1 coenzyme (TPP) is involved in

(a) Oxidative decarboxylation (b) Hydroxylation

(c) Transamination (d) Carboxylation

60. Increased glucose consumption increases the dietary requirement for

(a) Pyridoxine (b) Niacin

(c) Biotin (d) Thiamin

Answers

1	(a)	16	(c)	31	(d)	46	(c)
2	(b)	17	(a)	32	(a)	47	(a)
3	(a)	18	(a)	33	(c)	48	(c)
4	(a)	19	(a)	34	(c)	49	(b)
5	(a)	20	(a)	35	(b)	50	(a)
6	(a)	21	(b)	36	(a)	51	(d)
7	(d)	22	(d)	37	(c)	52	(c)
8	(a)	23	(a)	38	(b)	53	(c)
9	(d)	24	(c)	39	(a)	54	(c)
10	(a)	25	(c)	40	(d)	55	(d)
11	(b)	26	(a)	41	(d)	56	(b)
12	(b)	27	(a)	42	(d)	57	(c)
13	(a)	28	(a)	43	(a)	58	(a)
14	(d)	29	(c)	44	(a)	59	(a)
15	(b)	30	(a)	45	(b)	60	(d)

Chapter 18
Amino Acid Metabolism

1. **Oxidative deamination is the conversion of an amino**
   (a) Group from an amino acid to a keto acid
   (b) Acid to a carboxylic acid plus ammonia
   (c) Acid to a keto acid plus ammonia
   (d) Group from an amino acid to a carboxylic acid
2. **Transamination is the transfer of an amino**
   (a) Acid to a carboxylic acid plus ammonia
   (b) Group from an amino acid to a keto acid
   (c) Acid to a keto acid plus ammonia
   (d) Group from an amino acid to a carboxylic acid
3. **Transamination is the process where**
   (a) Carboxyl group is transferred from amino acid
   (b) A-amino group is removed from the amino acid
   (c) Polymerisation of amino acid takes place
   (d) None of the above
4. **Transaminase enzymes are present in**
   (a) Liver
   (b) Intestine
   (c) Pancreas
   (d) None of these
5. **An example of the oxidative deamination is**
   (a) Glutamate = hexanoic acid + NH_3
   (b) Aspartate + a-ketoglutarate = glutamate + oxaloacetate
   (c) Glutamate = a-ketoglutarate + NH_3
   (d) Aspartate + hexanoic acid = glutamate + Oxaloacetate

6. **A ketogenic amino acid is one which degrades to**
   (a) Keto-sugars
   (b) Either acetyl CoA or acetoacetyl CoA
   (c) Pyruvate or citric acid cycle intermediates
   (d) Multiple intermediates including pyruvate or citric acid cycle intermediates and acetyl CoA or acetoacetyl CoA

7. **A glucogenic amino acid is one which is degraded to**
   (a) Keto-sugars
   (b) Either acetyl CoA or acetoacetyl CoA
   (c) Pyruvate or citric acid cycle intermediates
   (d) None of the above

8. **A best described ketogenic amino acid is**
   (a) Lysine (b) Tryptophan
   (c) Valine (d) None of these

9. **Which of the following is the best described glucogenic amino acid?**
   (a) Lysine (b) Tryptophan
   (c) Valine (d) None of these

10. **Which of the following amino acids is considered as both ketogenic and glucogenic?**
   (a) Valine (b) Tryptophan
   (c) Lysine (d) None of these

11. **Lysine is degraded to acetoacetyl CoA and is described as a**
   (a) Ketogenic amino acid (b) Glucogenic amino acid
   (c) Keto-gluco amino acid (d) None of these

12. **Histidine is degraded to a-ketoglutarate and is described as a**
   (a) Glucogenic amino acid (b) Glucogenic amino acid
   (c) Ketogenic amino acid (d) Keto-gluco amino acid

13. **Tyrosine is degraded to acetoacetyl CoA and fumarate and is described as a**
   (a) Glucogenic amino acid (b) Ketogenic amino acid
   (c) Ketogenic and glucogenic amino acid (d) Keto-gluco amino acid

14. **In the normal breakdown of phenylalanine, it is initially degraded to**
   (a) Fumarate (b) Tryrosine
   (c) Lysine (d) Phenylpuruvate

15. A person with phenylketonuria cannot convert

(a) Phenylalanine to tyrosine
(b) Phenylalanine to isoleucine
(c) Phenol into ketones
(d) Phenylalanine to lysine

16. A person with phenylketonuria will convert

(a) Phenylalanine to phenylpyruvate
(b) Phenylalanine to isoleucine
(c) Phenylpyruvate to phenylalanine
(d) Tyrosine to phenylalanine

17. The most toxic compounds is

(a) Tyrosine
(b) Phenylpyruvate
(c) Lysine
(d) Phenylalanine

18. A person with phenylketonuria is advised not to consume which of the following products?

(a) Glycine containing foods
(b) Fat containing food
(c) Glucose
(d) Aspartame

19. A person suffering from phenylketonuria on consumption food containing high phenylalanine may lead to the accumulation of

(a) Phenylalanine
(b) Phenylpyruvate
(c) Tyrosine
(d) Isoleucine

20. An example of a transamination process is

(a) Glutamate = hexanoic acid + NH_3
(b) Aspartate + hexanoic acid = glutamate + oxaloacetate
(c) Aspartate + a ketoglutarate = glutamate + oxaloacetate
(d) Glutamate = a-ketoglutarate + NH_3

Answers

1	(c)	6	(b)	11	(a)	16	(c)
2	(b)	7	(c)	12	(b)	17	(b)
3	(b)	8	(a)	13	(c)	18	(d)
4	(a)	9	(c)	14	(b)	19	(b)
5	(c)	10	(b)	15	(a)	20	(c)

Chapter 19
Fats and Fatty Acid Metabolism

1. **An example of a hydroxy fatty acid is**
   (a) Ricinoleic acid (b) Crotonic acid
   (c) Butyric acid (d) Oleic acid

2. **An example of a saturated fatty acid is**
   (a) Palmitic acid (b) Oleic acid
   (c) Linoleic acid (d) Erucic acid

3. **If the fatty acid is esterified with an alcohol of high molecular weight instead of glycerol, the resulting compound is**
   (a) Lipositol (b) Plasmalogen
   (c) Wax (d) Cephalin

4. **A fatty acid which is not synthesized in the body and has to be supplied in the diet is**
   (a) Palmitic acid (b) Lauric acid
   (c) Linolenic acid (d) Palmitoleic acid

5. **Essential fatty acid**
   (a) Linoleic acid (b) Linolenic acid
   (c) Arachidonic acid (d) All of these

6. **The fatty acid present in cerebrosides is**
   (a) Lignoceric acid (b) Valeric acid
   (c) Caprylic acid (d) Behenic acid

7. **The number of double bonds in arachidonic acid is**
   (a) 1 (b) 2
   (c) 4 (d) 6

8. **In humans a dietary essential fatty acid is**
   (a) Palmitic acid (b) Stearic acid
   (c) Oleic acid (d) Linoleic acid

9. **A lipid containing alcoholic amine residue is**
   (a) Phosphatidic acid (b) Ganglioside
   (c) Glucocerebroside (d) Sphingomyelin

10. **Cephalin consists of**
    (a) Glycerol, fatty acids, phosphoric acid and choline
    (b) Glycerol, fatty acids, phosphoric acid and ethanolamine
    (c) Glycerol, fatty acids, phosphoric acid and inositol
    (d) Glycerol, fatty acids, phosphoric acid and serine

11. **In mammals, the major fat in adipose tissues is**
    (a) Phospholipid (b) Cholesterol
    (c) Sphingolipids (d) Triacylglycerol

12. **Glycosphingolipids are a combination of**
    (a) Ceramide with one or more sugar residues
    (b) Glycerol with galactose
    (c) Sphingosine with galactose
    (d) Sphingosine with phosphoric acid

13. **The importance of phospholipids as constituent of cell membrane is because they possess**
    (a) Fatty acids
    (b) Both polar and nonpolar groups
    (c) Glycerol
    (d) Phosphoric acid

14. **In neutral fats, the unsaponificable matter includes**
    (a) Hydrocarbons (b) Triacylglycerol
    (c) Phospholipids (d) Cholsesterol

15. **Higher alcohol present in waxes is**
    (a) Benzyl (b) Methyl
    (c) Ethyl (d) Cetyl

16. **Kerasin consists of**
    (a) Nervonic acid (b) Lignoceric acid
    (c) Cervonic acid (d) Clupanodonic acid

17. Gangliosides are complex glycosphingolipids found in

(a) Liver (b) Brain

(c) Kidney (d) Muscle

18. Unsaturated fatty acid found in the cod liver oil and containing 5 double bonds is

(a) Clupanodonic acid (b) Cervonic acid

(c) Elaidic acid (d) Timnodonic acid

19. Phospholipid acting as surfactant is

(a) Cephalin (b) Phosphatidyl inositol

(c) Lecithin (d) Phosphatidyl serine

20. An oil which contains cyclic fatty acids and once used in the treatment of leprosy is

(a) Elaidic oil (b) Rapeseed oil

(c) Lanoline (d) Chaulmoogric oil

21. Unpleasant odours and taste in a fat (rancidity) can be delayed or prevented by the addition of

(a) Lead (b) Copper

(c) Tocopherol (d) Ergosterol

22. Gangliosides derived from glucosylceramide contain in addition one or more molecules of

(a) Sialic acid (b) Glycerol

(c) Diacylglycerol (d) Hyaluronic acid

23. 'Drying oil', oxidized spontaneously by atmospheric oxygen at ordinary temperature and forms a hard water proof material is

(a) Coconut oil (b) Peanut oil

(c) Rape seed oil (d) Linseed oil

24. Deterioration of food (rancidity) is due to presence of

(a) Cholesterol (b) Vitamin E

(c) Peroxidation of lipids (d) Phenolic compounds

25. The number of ml of N/10 KOH required to neutralize the fatty acids in the distillate from 5 gm of fat is called

(a) Reichert-Meissel number

(b) Polenske number

(c) Acetyl number

(d) Non volatile fatty acid number

26. Molecular formula of cholesterol is

(a) $C_{27}H_{45}OH$ (b) $C_{29}H_{47}OH$

(c) $C_{29}H_{47}OH$ (d) $C_{23}H_{41}OH$

27. The cholesterol molecule is

(a) Benzene derivative (b) Quinoline derivative

(c) Steroid (d) Straight chain acid

28. Salkowski test is performed to detect

(a) Glycerol (b) Cholesterol

(c) Fatty acids (d) Vitamin D

29. Palmitic, oleic or stearic acid ester of cholesterol used 30. Dietary fats after absorption appear in the circulation as

(a) HDL (b) VLDL

(c) LDL (d) Chylomicron

31. Free fatty acids are transported in the blood

(a) Combined with albumin

(b) Combined with fatty acid binding protein

(c) Combined with β-lipoprotein

(d) In unbound free salts

32. Long chain fatty acids are first activated to acetyl-CoA in

(a) Cytosol (b) Microsomes

(c) Nucleus (d) Mitochondria

33. The enzyme acyl-CoA synthase catalyses the conversion of a fatty acid of an active fatty acid in the presence of

(a) AMP (b) ADP

(c) ATP (d) GTP

34. Carnitine is synthesized from

(a) Lysine and methionine (b) Glycine and arginine

(c) Aspartate and glutamate (d) Proline and hydroxyproline

35. The enzymes of β-oxidation are found in

(a) Mitochondria (b) Cytosol

(c) Golgi apparatus (d) Nucleus

36. Long chain fatty acids penetrate the inner mitochondrial membrane

(a) Requiring Na dependent carrier (b) As acyl-CoA derivative

(c) As carnitine derivative (d) Freely

37. An important feature of Zellweger's syndrome is

(a) Hypoglycemia
(b) Accumulation of phytanic acid in tissues
(c) Skin eruptions
(d) Accumulation of C26-C38 polyenoic acid in brain tissues

38. An important finding of Fabry's disease is

(a) Skin rash (b) Exophthalmos
(c) Hemolytic anemia (d) Mental retardation

39. Gaucher's disease is due to deficiency of the enzyme:

(a) Sphingomyelinase (b) Glucocerebrosidase
(c) Galactocerbrosidase (d) α-Galactosidase

40. Characteristic finding in Gaucher's disease is

(a) Night blindness (b) Renal failure
(c) Hepatosplenomegaly (d) Deafness

41. An important finding in Neimann-Pick disease is

(a) Leukopenia (b) Cardiac enlargement
(c) Corneal opacity (d) Hepatosplenomegaly

42. Fucosidosis is characterized by

(a) Muscle spasticity (b) Liver enlargement
(c) Skin rash (d) Kidney failure

43. Metachromatic leukodystrophy is due to deficiency of enzyme

(a) α-fucosidase (b) Arylsulphatase A
(c) Ceramidase (d) Hexosaminidase A

44. A significant feature of Tangier disease is

(a) Impairment of chylomicron formation (b) Hypotriacylglycerolmia
(c) Absence of Apo-C-II (d) Absence of Apo-C-I

45. A significant feature of Broad Beta disease is

(a) Hypocholesterolemia (b) Hypotriacylglycerolemia
(c) Absence of Apo-D (d) Abnormality of Apo-E

46. Neonatal tyrosinemia improves on administration of

(a) Thiamin (b) Riboflavin
(c) Pyridoxine (d) Ascorbic acid

47. Absence of phenylalanine hydroxylase causes
(a) Neonatal tyrosinemia (b) Phenylketonuria
(c) Primary hyperoxaluria (d) Albinism

48. Richner-Hanhart syndrome is due to defect in
(a) Fumarylacetoacetate hydrolase (b) Phenylalanine hydroxylase
(c) Hepatic tyrosine transaminase (d) Tyrosinase

49. Plasma tyrosine level in Richner-Hanhart syndrome is
(a) 1–2 mg/dL (b) 2–3 mg/dL
(c) 4–5 mg/dL (d) 8–10 mg/dL

50. Amount of phenylacetic acid excreted in the urine in phenylketonuria is
(a) 100–200 mg/dL (b) 200–280 mg/dL
(c) 290–550 mg/dL (d) 600–750 mg/dL

51. Tyrosinosis is due to defect in the enzyme
(a) Fumarylacetoacetate hydrolase
(b) p-Hydroxyphenylpyruvate hydroxylase
(c) Tyrosine transaminase
(d) Tyrosine hydroxylase

52. An important finding in Histidinemia is
(a) Impairment of conversion of α-glutamate to α-ketoglutarate
(b) Speech defect
(c) Decreased urinary histidine level
(d) Patients can not be treated by diet

53. An important finding in glycinuria is
(a) Excess excretion of oxalate in the urine
(b) Deficiency of enzyme glycinase
(c) Significantly increased serum glycine level
(d) Defect in renal tubular reabsorption of glycine

54. Increased urinary indole acetic acid is diagnostic of
(a) Maple syrup urine disease (b) Hartnup disease
(c) Homocystinuia (d) Phenylketonuria

55. In glycinuria daily urinary excretion of glycine ranges from
(a) 100–200 mg (b) 300–500 mg
(c) 600–1000 mg (d) 1100–1400 mg

56. An inborn error, maple syrup urine disease is due to deficiency of the enzyme

(a) Isovaleryl-CoAhydrogenase (b) Phenylalnine hydroxylase

(c) Adenosyl transferase (d) α-Ketoacid decarboxylase

57. Maple syrup urine disease becomes evident in extra uterine life by the end of

(a) First week (b) Second week

(c) Third week (d) Fourth week

58. Alkaptonuria occurs due to deficiency of the enzyme:

(a) Maleylacetoacetate isomerase

(b) Homogentisate oxidase

(c) p-Hydroxyphenylpyruvate hydroxylase

(d) Fumarylacetoacetate hydrolase

59. An important feature of maple syrup urine disease is

(a) Patient can not be treated by dietary regulation

(b) Without treatment death, of patient may occur by the end of second year of life

(c) Blood levels of leucine, isoleucine and serine are increased

(d) Excessive brain damage

60. Ochronosis is an important finding of

(a) Tyrosinemia (b) Tyrosinosis

(c) Alkaptonuria (d) Richner Hanhart syndrome

Answers

1	(a)	16	(b)	31	(a)	46	(a)
2	(a)	17	(b)	32	(a)	47	(d)
3	(c)	18	(d)	33	(c)	48	(b)
4	(c)	19	(c)	34	(a)	49	(c)
5	(d)	20	(d)	35	(a)	50	(c)
6	(a)	21	(c)	36	(c)	51	(a)
7	(c)	22	(a)	37	(d)	52	(b)
8	(d)	23	(d)	38	(a)	53	(d)
9	(d)	24	(c)	39	(b)	54	(b)
10	(b)	25	(a)	40	(c)	55	(c)
11	(d)	26	(a)	41	(d)	56	(d)
12	(a)	27	(c)	42	(a)	57	(a)
13	(b)	28	(b)	43	(b)	58	(b)
14	(a)	29	(b)	44	(c)	59	(d)
15	(d)	30	(d)	45	(d)	60	(c)

Chapter 20
Enzymes

1. **The compound which has the lowest density is**
   (a) Chylomicron
   (b) α-lipoprotein
   (c) β-lipoprotein
   (d) Pre α-lipoprotein

2. **Non steroidal anti inflammatory drugs, such as aspirin act by inhibiting the activity of the enzyme**
   (a) Lipoxygenase
   (b) Cyclooxygenase
   (c) Phospholipase A2
   (d) Lipoprotein lipase

3. **From arachidonate, synthesis of prostaglandins is catalysed by**
   (a) Cyclooxygenase
   (b) Lipoxygenase
   (c) Thromboxane synthase
   (d) Isomerase

4. **A Holoenzyme is**
   (a) Functional unit
   (b) Apo enzyme
   (c) Coenzyme
   (d) All of these

5. **Gaucher's disease is due to the deficiency of the enzyme**
   (a) α-fucosidase
   (b) α-galactosidase
   (c) β-glucosidase
   (d) Sphingomyelinase

6. **Neimann-Pick disease is due to the deficiency of the enzyme**
   (a) Hexosaminidase A and B
   (b) Ceramidase
   (c) Ceramide lactosidase
   (d) Sphingomyelinase

7. **Krabbe's disease is due to the deficiency of the enzyme**
   (a) Ceramide lactosidase
   (b) Ceramidase
   (c) β-galactosidase
   (d) GM1 β-galactosidase

8. **Fabry's disease is due to the deficiency of the enzyme**
   (a) Ceramide trihexosidase
   (b) Galactocerebrosidase
   (c) Phytanic acid oxidase
   (d) Sphingomyelinase

9. **Farber's disease is due to the deficiency of the enzyme**
   (a) β-galactosidase (b) Ceramidase
   (c) β-glucocerebrosidase (d) Arylsulphatase A.

10. **A synthetic nucleotide analogue, used in organ transplantation as a suppressor of immunologic rejection of grafts is**
   (a) Theophylline (b) Cytarabine
   (c) 4-Hydroxypyrazolopyrimidine (d) 6-Mercaptopurine

11. **Example of an extracellular enzyme is**
   (a) Lactate dehydrogenase (b) Cytochrome oxidase
   (c) Pancreatic lipase (d) Hexokinase

12. **Enzymes, which are produced in inactive form in the living cells, are called**
   (a) Papain (b) Lysozymes
   (c) Apoenzymes (d) Proenzymes

13. **An example of ligases is**
   (a) Succinate thiokinase (b) Alanine racemase
   (c) Fumarase (d) Aldolase

14. **An example of lyases is**
   (a) Glutamine synthetase (b) Fumarase
   (c) Cholinesterase (d) Amylase

15. **Activation or inactivation of certain key regulatory enzymes is accomplished by covalent modification of the amino acid:**
   (a) Tyrosine (b) Phenylalanine
   (c) Lysine (d) Serine

16. **The enzyme which can add water to a carbon-carbon double bond or remove water to create a double bond without breaking the bond is**
   (a) Hydratase (b) Hydroxylase
   (c) Hydrolase (d) Esterase

17. **Fischer's 'lock and key' model of the enzyme action implies that**
   (a) The active site is complementary in shape to that of substance only after interaction
   (b) The active site is complementary in shape to that of substance
   (c) Substrates change conformation prior to active site interaction
   (d) The active site is flexible and adjusts to substrate

18. From the Lineweaver-Burk plot of Michaelis-Menten equation, Km and Vmax can be determined when V is the reaction velocity at substrate concentration S, the X-axis experimental data are expressed as

(a) 1/V (b) V

(c) 1/S (d) S

19. A sigmoidal plot of substrate concentration ([S]) verses reaction velocity (V) may indicate

(a) Michaelis-Menten kinetics (b) Co-operative binding

(c) Competitive inhibition (d) Non-competitive inhibition

20. The Km of the enzyme giving the kinetic data as below is

(a) –0.50 (b) –0.25

(c) +0.25 (d) +0.33

21. The kinetic effect of purely competitive inhibitor of an enzyme

(a) Increases Km without affecting Vmax

(b) Decreases Km without affecting Vmax

(c) Increases Vmax without affecting Km

(d) Decreases Vmax without affecting Km

22. If curve X in the graph (below) represents no inhibition for the reaction of the enzyme with its substrates, the curve representing the competitive inhibition, of the same reaction is

(a) A (b) B

(c) C (d) D

23. An inducer is absent in the type of enzyme

(a) Allosteric enzyme (b) Constitutive enzyme

(c) Co-operative enzyme (d) Isoenzymic enzyme

24. A demonstrable inducer is absent in

(a) Allosteric enzyme (b) Constitutive enzyme

(c) Inhibited enzyme (d) Co-operative enzyme

25. In reversible non-competitive enzyme activity inhibition

(a) Vmax is increased

(b) Km is increased

(c) Km is decreased

(d) Concentration of active enzyme is reduced

26. In reversible non-competitive enzyme activity inhibition

(a) Inhibitor bears structural resemblance to substrate

(b) Inhibitor lowers the maximum velocity attainable with a given amount of enzyme

(c) Km is increased

(d) Km is decreased

27. In competitive enzyme activity inhibition

(a) The structure of inhibitor generally resembles that of the substrate

(b) Inhibitor decreases apparent Km

(c) Km remains unaffective

(d) Inhibitor decreases Vmax without affecting Km

28. In enzyme kinetics Vmax reflects

(a) The amount of an active enzyme (b) Substrate concentration

(c) Half the substrate concentration (d) Enzyme substrate complex

29. In enzyme kinetics Km implies

(a) The substrate concentration that gives one half Vmax

(b) The dissocation constant for the enzyme substrate comples

(c) Concentration of enzyme

(d) Half of the substrate concentration required to achieve Vmax

30. In competitive enzyme activity inhibition

(a) Apparent Km is decreased (b) Apparent Km is increased

(c) Vmax is increased (d) Vmax is decreased

31. In non competitive enzyme activity inhibition, inhibitor

(a) Increases Km (b) Decreases Km

(c) Does not effect Km (d) Increases Km

32. An enzyme catalyzing oxidoreduction, using oxygen as hydrogen acceptor is

(a) Cytochrome oxidase (b) Lactate dehydrogenase

(c) Malate dehydrogenase (d) Succinate dehydrogenase

33. The enzyme using some other substance, not oxygen as hydrogen acceptor is

(a) Tyrosinase (b) Succinate dehydrogenase

(c) Uricase (d) Cytochrome oxidase

34. An enzyme which uses hydrogen acceptor as substrate is

(a) Xanthine oxidase (b) Aldehyde oxidase

(c) Catalase (d) Tryptophan oxygenase

35. **Enzyme involved in joining together two substrates is**
(a) Glutamine synthetase (b) Aldolase
(c) Gunaine deaminase (d) Arginase

36. **The pH optima of most of the enzymes is**
(a) Between 2 and 4 (b) Between 5 and 9
(c) Between 8 and 12 (d) Above 12

37. **Coenzymes are**
(a) Heat stable, dialyzable, non protein organic molecules
(b) Soluble, colloidal, protein molecules
(c) Structural analogue of enzymes
(d) Different forms of enzymes

38. **An example of hydrogen transferring coenzyme is**
(a) CoA (b) NAD+
(c) Biotin (d) TPP

39. **An example of group transferring coenzyme is**
(a) NAD+ (b) NADP+
(c) FAD (d) CoA

40. **Cocarboxylase is**
(a) Thiamine pyrophosphate (b) Pyridoxal phosphate
(c) Biotin (d) CoA

41. **A coenzyme containing non aromatic hetero ring is**
(a) ATP (b) NAD
(c) FMN (d) Biotin

42. **A coenzyme containing aromatic hetero ring is**
(a) TPP (b) Lipoic acid
(c) Coenzyme Q (d) Biotin

43. **Isoenzymes are**
(a) Chemically, immunologically and electrophoretically different forms of an enzyme
(b) Different forms of an enzyme similar in all properties
(c) Catalysing different reactions
(d) Having the same quaternary structures like the enzymes

44. Isoenzymes can be characterized by

(a) Proteins lacking enzymatic activity that are necessary for the activation of enzymes

(b) Proteolytic enzymes activated by hydrolysis

(c) Enzymes with identical primary structure

(d) Similar enzymes that catalyse different reaction

45. The isoenzymes of LDH

(a) Differ only in a single amino acid

(b) Differ in catalytic activity

(c) Exist in 5 forms depending on M and H monomer contents

(d) Occur as monomers

46. The normal value of CPK in serum varies between

(a) 4–60 IU/L (b) 60–250 IU/L

(c) 4–17 IU/L (d) > 350 IU/L

47. Factors affecting enzyme activity

(a) Concentration (b) pH

(c) Temperature (d) All of these

48. The normal serum GOT activity ranges from

(a) 3.0–15.0 IU/L (b) 4.0–17.0 IU/

(c) 4.0–60.0 IU/L (d) 0.9–4.0 IU/L

49. The normal GPT activity ranges from

(a) 60.0–250.0 IU/L (b) 4.0–17.0 IU/L

(c) 3.0–15.0 IU/L (d) 0.1–14.0 IU/L

50. The normal serum acid phosphatase activity ranges from

(a) 5.0–13.0 KA units/100 ml (b) 1.0–5.0 KA units/100 ml

(c) 13.0–18.0 KA units/100 ml (d) 0.2–0.8 KA units/100 ml

Answers

1	(a)	14	(b)	27	(a)	40	(c)
2	(b)	15	(d)	28	(a)	41	(d)
3	(a)	16	(a)	29	(a)	42	(a)
4	(d)	17	(b)	30	(b)	43	(a)
5	(c)	18	(c)	31	(c)	44	(b)
6	(d)	19	(b)	32	(a)	45	(c)
7	(c)	20	(d)	33	(b)	46	(a)
8	(a)	21	(a)	34	(c)	47	(d)
9	(b)	22	(a)	35	(a)	48	(b)
10	(d)	23	(b)	36	(b)	49	(c)
11	(c)	24	(b)	37	(a)	50	(b)
12	(d)	25	(d)	38	(b)		
13	(a)	26	(b)	39	(d)		

Chapter 21
Nucleic Acids

1. **A nucleoside consists of**
   (a) Nitrogenous base
   (b) Purine or pyrimidine base + sugar
   (c) Purine or pyrimidine base + phosphorus
   (d) Purine + pyrimidine base + sugar + phosphorus

2. **A nucleotide consists of**
   (a) A nitrogenous base like choline
   (b) Purine + pyrimidine base + sugar + phosphorus
   (c) Purine or pyrimidine base + sugar
   (d) Purine or pyrimidine base + phosphorus

3. **A purine nucleotide is**
   (a) AMP (b) UMP
   (c) CMP (d) TMP

4. **A pyrimidine nucleotide is**
   (a) GMP (b) AMP
   (c) CMP (d) IMP

5. **Adenine is**
   (a) 6-Amino purine (b) 2-Amino-6-oxypurine
   (c) 2-Oxy-4-aminopyrimidine (d) 2, 4-Dioxypyrimidine

6. **2, 4-Dioxypyrimidine is**
   (a) Thymine (b) Cystosine
   (c) Uracil (d) Guanine

7. **The chemical name of guanine is**
   (a) 2,4-Dioxy-5-methylpyrimidine (b) 2-Amino-6-oxypurine
   (c) 2-Oxy-4-aminopyrimidine (d) 2, 4-Dioxypyrimidine

8. **Nucleotides and nucleic acids concentration are often also expressed in terms of**
   (a) Ng (b) Mg
   (c) Meq (d) OD at 260 nm

9. **The pyrimidine nucleotide acting as the high energy intermediate is**
   (a) ATP (b) UTP
   (c) UDPG (d) CMP

10. **The carbon of the pentose in ester linkage with the phosphate in a nucleotide structure is**
    (a) C1 (b) C3
    (c) C4 (d) C5

11. **Uracil and ribose form**
    (a) Uridine (b) Cytidine
    (c) Guanosine (d) Adenosine

12. **The most abundant free nucleotide in mammalian cells is**
    (a) ATP (b) NAD
    (c) GTP (d) FAD

13. **The mean intracellular concentration of ATP in mammalian cell is about**
    (a) 1 mM (b) 2 mM
    (c) 0.1 mM (d) 0.2 mM

14. **The nucleic acid base found in mRNA but not in DNA is**
    (a) Adenine (b) Cytosine
    (c) Guanine (d) Uracil

15. **In RNA moleule 'Caps'**
    (a) Allow tRNA to be processed
    (b) Are unique to eukaryotic mRNA
    (c) Occur at the 3′ end of tRNA
    (d) Allow correct translation of prokaryotic mRNA

16. **In contrast to eukaryotic mRNA, prokaryotic mRNA**
    (a) Can be polycistronic (b) Is synthesized with introns
    (c) Can only be monocistronic (d) Has a poly A tail

17. **The size of small stable RNA ranges from**
    (a) 0–40 nucleotides (b) 40–80 nucleotides
    (c) 90–300 nucleotides (d) More than 320 nucleotides

18. The number of small stable RNAs per cell ranges from

(a) 10–50,000 (b) 50,000–1,00,000

(c) 1,00,000–10,00,000 (d) More than 10 lakhs

19. Molecular weight of heterogenous nuclear RNA (hnRNA) is

(a) More than 107 (b) 105 to 106

(c) 104 to 105 (d) Less than 104

20. In RNA molecule guanine content does not necessarily equal its cytosine content nor does its adenine content necessarily equal its uracil content since it is a

(a) Single strand molecule

(b) Double stranded molecule

(c) Double stranded helical molecule

(d) Polymer of purine and pyrimidine ribonucleotides

21. The nitrogenous base present in the RNA molecule is

(a) Thymine (b) Uracil

(c) Xanthine (d) Hypoxanthine

22. RNA does not contain

(a) Uracil (b) Adenine

(c) Thymine (d) Ribose

23. The sugar moiety present in RNA is

(a) Ribulose (b) Arabinose

(c) Ribose (d) Dcoxyribose

24. In RNA molecule

(a) Guanine content equals cytosine

(b) Adenine content equals uracil

(c) Adenine content equals guanine

(d) Guanine content does not necessarily equal its cytosine content

25. Methylated purines and pyrimidines are characteristically present in

(a) *m*RNA (b) *h*nRNA

(c) *t*RNA (d) *r*RNA

26. Thymine is present in

(a) *t*RNA (b) Ribosomal RNA

(c) Mammalian mRNA (d) Prokaryotic *m*RNA

27. The approximate number of nucleotides in tRNA molecule is

(a) 25 (b) 50
(c) 75 (d) 100

28. In every cell, the number of tRNA molecules is at least

(a) 10 (b) 20
(c) 30 (d) 40

29. The structure of tRNA appears like a

(a) Helix (b) Hair pin
(c) Clover leaf (d) Coil

30. Although each specific tRNA differs from the others in its sequence of nucleotides, all tRNA molecules contain a base paired stem that terminates in the sequence CCA at

(a) 32 Termini (b) 52 Termini
(c) Anticodon arm (d) 3252 Termini

31. Transfer RNAs are classified on the basis of the number of base pairs in

(a) Acceptor arm (b) Anticodon arm
(c) D arm (d) Extra arm

32. In tRNA molecule D arm is named for the presence of the base

(a) Uridine (b) Pseudouridine
(c) Dihydrouridine (d) Thymidine

33. The acceptor arm in the tRNA molecule has

(a) 5 Base pairs (b) 7 Base pairs
(c) 10 Base pairs (d) 20 Base pairs

34. In tRNA molecule, the anticodon arm possesses

(a) 5 Base pairs (b) 7 Base pairs
(c) 8 Base pairs (d) 10 Base pairs

35. The T ??C arm in the tRNA molecule possesses the sequence

(a) T, pseudouridine and C (b) T, uridine and C
(c) T, dihydrouridine and C (d) T, adenine and C

36. Double helical structure model of the DNA was proposed by

(a) Pauling and Corey (b) Peter Mitchell
(c) Watson and Crick (d) King and Wooten

37. DNA does not contain

(a) Thymine (b) Adenine

(c) Uracil (d) Deoxyribose

38. The sugar moiety present in DNA is

(a) Deoxyribose (b) Ribose

(c) Lyxose (d) Ribulose

39. DNA rich in A-T pairs have

(a) 1 Hydrogen bond (b) 2 Hydrogen bonds

(c) 3 Hydrogen bonds (d) 4 Hydrogen bonds

40. In DNA molecule

(a) Guanine content does not equal cytosine content

(b) Adenine content does not equal thymine content

(c) Adenine content equals uracil content

(d) Guanine content equals cytosine content

41. DNA rich in G-C pairs have

(a) 1 Hydrogen bond (b) 2 Hydrogen bonds

(c) 3 Hydrogen bonds (d) 4 Hydrogen bonds

42. The fact that DNA bears the genetic information of an organism implies that

(a) Base composition should be identical from species to species

(b) DNA base composition should charge with age

(c) DNA from different tissues in the same organism should usually have the same base composition

(d) DNA base composition is altered with nutritional state of an organism

43. The width (helical diameter) of the double helix in B-form DNA in nm is

(a) 1 (b) 2

(c) 3 (d) 4

44. The number of base pair in a single turn of B-form DNA about the axis of the molecule is

(a) 4 (b) 8

(c) 10 (d) 12

45. The distance spanned by one turn of B-form DNA is

(a) 1.0 nm (b) 2.0 nm

(c) 3.0 nm (d) 3.4 nm

46. In a DNA molecule the thymine concentration is 30 per cent , the guanosine concentration will be

(a) 10 per cent (b) 20 per cent
(c) 30 per cent (d) 40 per cent

47. IN a DNA molecule, the guanosine content is 40 per cent , the adenine content will be

(a) 10 per cent (b) 20 per cent
(c) 30 per cent (d) 40 per cent

48. An increased melting temperature of duplex DNA results from a high content of

(a) Adenine + Guanine (b) Thymine + Cytosine
(c) Cytosine + Guanine (d) Cytosine + Adenine

49. A synthetic nucleotide analogue, 4-hydroxypyrazolopyrimidine is used in the treatment of

(a) Acute nephritis (b) Gout
(c) Cystic fibrosis of lung (d) Multiple myeloma

50. A synthetic nucleotide analogue, used in the chemotherapy of cancer and viral infections is

(a) Arabinosyl cytosine (b) 6-Mercaptopurine
(c) 4-Hydroxypyrazolopyrimidine (d) 6-Thioguanine

Answers

1	(b)	14	(d)	27	(c)	40	(d)
2	(b)	15	(b)	28	(b)	41	(c)
3	(a)	16	(a)	29	(c)	42	(c)
4	(c)	17	(c)	30	(a)	43	(b)
5	(a)	18	(c)	31	(d)	44	(c)
6	(c)	19	(a)	32	(a)	45	(d)
7	(b)	20	(a)	33	(b)	46	(b)
8	(d)	21	(b)	34	(a)	47	(a)
9	(c)	22	(c)	35	(a)	48	(c)
10	(d)	23	(c)	36	(c)	49	(b)
11	(a)	24	(d)	37	(c)	50	(a)
12	(a)	25	(c)	38	(a)		
13	(a)	26	(a)	39	(b)		

Chapter 22
Plant Biotechnology

Plant: General

1. **Who among the following coined the term Biotechnology?**
   (a) Karl Ereky
   (b) James Clarke
   (c) Paul Terasaky
   (d) Clarke and Sommer

2. **Triticale, the first man made cereal is an example of**
   (a) Artificial allopolyploidy
   (b) Artificial autopolyploidy
   (c) Man made crossing
   (d) Artificial evolution

3. **Triticale is derived by crossing**
   (a) Wheat and rice
   (b) Wheat and tapioca
   (c) Rye (secale) and wheat
   (d) Rye and rice

4. **In the bundle sheath of C4 plant is/ are less than mesophyll.**
   (a) PSI
   (b) PSII
   (c) PSI or PSII
   (d) PSI and PSII

5. **Rice can grow in water submerged soil because the plants**
   (a) Have spongy roots
   (b) Can oxidize the micro-environment around their roots and thus able to absorb oxygen
   (c) Are adapted to enable roots to ward off toxic products
   (d) All of the above

6. **Gypsum is beneficial for**
   (a) Phosphorus enriched soil
   (b) Water logged soil
   (c) Alkaline soil
   (d) Saline soil

7. **The volume of O_2 liberated in photosynthesis has which of the following ratio to CO_2?**
   (a) 1: 1 (b) 2:1
   (c) 1: 2 (d) 3:1

8. **The major source of sugar in the world is**
   (a) Watermelon (b) Beetroot
   (c) Sugarcane (d) Dates

9. **The study of interaction between living organism of environment is called**
   (a) Ecosystem (b) Phytogeography
   (c) Ecology (d) Photosociology

10. **Auxanometer is used for measuring**
    (a) Respiratory activity (b) Photosynthetic activity
    (c) Growth activity (d) Osmotic pressure

11. **The colour of flower is due to the presence of**
    (a) Chlorophyll (b) Xanthophylls
    (c) Florigen (d) Chromoplast or anthocyanin

12. **In angiosperm, the endosperm is**
    (a) Haploid (b) Diploid
    (c) Triploid (d) None of these

13. **Neurospora is used as an experimental tool in**
    (a) Ecology (b) Cytology
    (c) Genetics (d) Physiology

14. **Lichen involves two organisms as**
    (a) Virus and bacteria (b) Algae and bacteria
    (c) Algae and fungi (d) Fungi and mosses

15. **The proteins that forms the walls of the microtubules are**
    (a) Actin (b) Tubulin
    (c) Pectin (d) Hydroxyproline

16. **Archaeabacteria differ from the true bacteria as they have**
    (a) Different cell membrane lipids
    (b) Cell wall composition
    (c) Ribosomal RNA structure
    (d) Growth not inhibited by antibiotics

17. Which group of land plants is most restricted to moist environments?

(a) Lycophyta
(b) Sphenophyta
(c) Bryophyta
(d) Angiosperms

18. Which group of plants has the greatest diversity (*i.e.* the most species) living today?

(a) Bryophyta
(b) Lycophyta
(c) Gymnosperms
(d) Angiosperms

19. What single feature is probably most respon ible for the success of angiosperms?

(a) Seeds
(b) Fruit
(c) Broad leaves
(d) Flowers

20. A very common mutualistic, symbiotic relationship between a fungus and the roots of a plant is

(a) Lichen
(b) Mycorrhizal
(c) Ascomycete
(d) Basidiomycete

21. What are the names of the two genders of haploid yeast cells?

(a) A and Alpha
(b) M and F
(c) Y (a) and Y (b)
(d) None of these

22. Mycorrhizae are symbiotic associations between

(a) Algae and fungi
(b) Root and fungi
(c) Bacteria and root
(d) Bacteria and fungi

Answers

1	(a)	7	(a)	13	(c)	19	(d)
2	(a)	8	(b)	14	(c)	20	(b)
3	(c)	9	(c)	15	(b)	21	(a)
4	(b)	10	(c)	16	(b)	22	(b)
5	(d)	11	(d)	17	(c)		
6	(c)	12	(c)	18	(d)		

Chapter 23
Cloning Vectors

1. **Select the wrong statement about plasmids?**
   (a) It is extrachromosomal
   (b) It is double stranded
   (c) Its replication depends upon host cell
   (d) It is closed and circular DNA
2. **A plasmid can be considered as a suitable cloning vector if**
   (a) It can be readily isolated from the cells
   (b) It possesses a single restriction site for one or more restriction enzymes
   (c) Insertion of foreign DNA does not alter its replication properties
   (d) All of the above
3. **pBR 322 has/have which of the following selection marker(s)?**
   (a) Amp (b) Tetr
   (c) Both (a) and (b) (d) Kant
4. **Cosmids lack**
   (a) Genes coding for viral proteins
   (b) Origin of replication
   (c) Marker genes coding for replication
   (d) Cleavage site for the insertion of foreign DNA
5. **Cos site of the cosmids**
   (a) Consists of 12 bases
   (b) Helps whole genome in circularization and ligation
   (c) Both (a) and (b)
   (d) Contains cleavage site

6. **Size of the DNA that can be packaged into a X phage is**
   (a) 50 kb (b) 35-53 kb
   (c) 40-50 kb (d) Any size

7. **Maximum size of foreign DNA that can be inserted into an insertion vector is**
   (a) 35 kb (b) 18 kb
   (c) 50 kb (d) 27 kb

8. **Maximum size of foreign DNA that can be inserted into a replacement vector is**
   (a) 25-30 kb (b) 18-20 kb
   (c) 20-25 kb (d) 40-50 kb

9. **Cryptic plasmids**
   (a) Do not exhibit any phenotypic trait
   (b) Exhibit many phenotypic traits
   (c) Exhibit one phenotypic traits
   (d) Exhibit antibiotic resistance

10. **Plasmids which are maintained as multiple copy number per cell are known as**
    (a) Stringent plasmids (b) Relaxed plasmids
    (c) Cryptic plasmids (d) None of these.

11. **Plasmids which are maintained as limited number of copies per cell are known as**
    (a) Stringent plasmids (b) Relaxed plasmids
    (c) Cryptic plasmids (d) All of these.

12. **Conjugative plasmids**
    (a) Exhibit antibiotic resistance
    (b) Do not exhibit antibiotic resistance
    (c) Carry transfer genes called the tra genes
    (d) Do not carry transfer genes

13. **Plasmid incompatibility is**
    (a) Inability of a plasmid to grow in the host
    (b) Inability of two different plasmids to coexist in the same host cell in the absence of selection pressure
    (c) Both (a) and (b)
    (d) None of the above

14. Cosmid vectors are

(a) Plasmids that contain fragment of X DNA including the cos site

(b) Phages that lack cos site

(c) Plasmids that have no selection marker

(d) Cryptic plasmids

15. Cosmid vectors are used for

(a) Cloning small fragments of DNA

(b) Cloning large fragments of DNA

(c) Cloning prokaryotic DNA only

(d) Cloning eukaryotic DNA only

16. Phagemid vectors are

(a) Combination of plasmid and phage X

(b) Combination of phages and cosmid

(c) Phages carrying properties of plasmids

(d) All of the above

17. Phagemid consist of

(a) Plasmid vector carrying phage's cos site

(b) Plasmid vector carrying X attachment (X att) site

(c)

Plasmid vector carrying origin of replication of X phage only

(d) Plasmid vector carrying origin of replication of plasmid only

18. ZAP vector is an example of

(a) Phage (b) Phagemid

(c) Cosmid (d) Plasmid

19. Which of the following is not true about phagemid?

(a) Contain functional origin of replication of the plasmid and X phage

(b) May be propagated as a plasmid or as phage in appropriate strain

(c) Contain att site

(d) Can only be propagated as phage.

20. M 13 is an example of

(a) Filamentous phage (b) Single stranded DNA vector

(c) Both (a) and (b) (d) Plasmid

21. Single stranded vectors are useful

(a) For sequencing of cloned DNA

(b) For oligonucleotide directed mutagenesis

(c) For probe preparation

(d) All of the above

22. Difference between λ gt 10 and λ gt 11 vectors is that

(a) λ gt 11 is an expression vector

(b) λ gt 10 is an expression vector

(c) λ gt 10 is a replacement vector

(d) λ gt 11 is a replacement vector

23. Inserted DNA in λ gt 11 can be expressed as

(a) β-galactosidase fused protein

(b) Free protein in the cytoplasm

(c) Free protein that is secreted out

(d) All of the above

24. λ gt 10 and λ gt 11 vectors can propagate cloned fragments up to

(a) 6-7 kb

(b) 1-2 kb

(c) 40-44 kb

(d) 20-23 kb

25. EMBL 3 and EMBL 4 are replacement vectors, which can clone DNA up to

(a) 6-7 kb

(b) 15-25 kb

(c) 40-44 kb

(d) 1-2 kb

26. Stuffer is

(a) The right arm of the vector DNA

(b) The left arm of the vector DNA

(c) Central fragment of the vector DNA

(d) None of the above.

27. Charon 34 and Charon 35 are the examples of

(a) Plasmid vector

(b) Cosmid vector

(c) Phage vector

(d) Phagemid vector

28. Charon vectors are different from EMBL vectors because

(a) They have more extensive range of restriction targets with in their polylinkers

(b) Physical separation of lambda arm from central fragment is required

(c) Both (a) and (b)

(d) Physical separation of lambda arm from central fragment is not required

29. Charon 34 and Charon 35 can clone DNA upto

(a) 1-2 kb

(b) 6-7 kb

(c) 9-20 kb

(d) 30-35 kb

30. PI cloning vector is the example of

(a) Plasmid (b) Cosmid

(c) Bacteriophage (d) Phagemid

31. PI cloning vector allow cloning of DNA of the length of

(a) 100 kbp (b) 50 kbp

(c) 20 kbp (d) 10 kbp

Answers

1	(c)	9	(a)	17	(b)	25	(b)
2	(d)	10	(b)	18	(b)	26	(c)
3	(c)	11	(a)	19	(d)	27	(c)
4	(a)	12	(c)	20	(c)	28	(c)
5	(c)	13	(b)	21	(d)	29	(c)
6	(b)	14	(a)	22	(a)	30	(c)
7	(b)	15	(b)	23	(a)	31	(a)
8	(c)	16	(a)	24	(a)		

Chapter 24
Vector

1. **Maximum size of foreign DNA that can be inserted into a replacement vector is**
   (a) 25-30 kb
   (b) 18-20 kb
   (c) 20-25 kb
   (d) 40-50 kb

2. **Which of the following is not true about phagemid?**
   (a) Contain functional origin of replication of the plasmid and λ phage
   (b) May be propagated as a plasmid or as phage in appropriate strain
   (c) Contain λ site
   (d) Can only be propagated as phage

3. **pBR 322 has/have which of the following selection marker(s)?**
   (a) Amp^r
   (b) Tet^r
   (c) Both (a) and (b)
   (d) Kan^r

4. **A plasmid can be considered as a suitable cloning vector if**
   (a) It can be readily isolated from the cells
   (b) It possesses a single restriction site for one or more restriction enzymes
   (c) Insertion of foreign DNA does not alter its replication properties
   (d) All of the above

5. **Difference between λ gt 10 and λ gt 11 vectors is that**
   (a) λ gt 11 is an expression vector
   (b) λ gt 10 is an expression vector
   (c) λ gt 10 is a replacement vector
   (d) λ gt 11 is a replacement vector

6. **λ ZAP vector is an example of**
   (a) Phage
   (b) Phagemid
   (c) Cosmid
   (d) Plasmid

7. **λ gt 10 and λ gt 11 vectors can propagate cloned fragments up to**
   (a) 6-7 kb (b) 1-2 kb
   (c) 40-44 kb (d) 20-23 kb

8. **Select the wrong statement about plasmids?**
   (a) It is extrachromosomal (b) It is double stranded
   (c) Its replication depends upon host cell (d) It is closed and circular DNA

9. **Stuffer is**
   (a) The right arm of the vector DNA (b) The left arm of the vector DNA
   (c) Central fragment of the vector DNA (d) None of the above

10. **Conjugative plasmids**
    (a) Exhibit antibiotic resistance
    (b) Do not exhibit antibiotic resistance
    (c) Carry transfer genes called the *tra* genes
    (d) Do not carry transfer genes

11. **Plasmid incompatibility is**
    (a) Inability of a plasmid to grow in the host
    (b) Inability of two different plasmids to coexist in the same host cell in the absence of selection pressure.
    (c) Both (a) and (b)
    (d) None of the above

12. **P1 cloning vector allow cloning of DNA of the length of**
    (a) 100 kbp (b) 50 kbp
    (c) 20 kbp (d) 10 kbp

13. **Charon 34 and Charon 35 can clone DNA upto**
    (a) 1-2 kb (b) 6-7 kb
    (c) 9-20 kb (d) 30-35 kb

14. **Charon vectors are different from EMBL vectors because**
    (a) They have more extensive range of restriction targets with in their polylinkers
    (b) Physical separation of lambda arm from central fragment is required
    (c) Both (a) and (b)
    (d) Physical separation of lambda arm from central fragment is not required

15. **P1 cloning vector is the example of**
    (a) Plasmid (b) Cosmid
    (c) Bacteriophage (d) Phagemid

16. Cos site of the cosmids

(a) Consists of 12 bases

(b) Helps whole genome in circularization and ligation

(c) Both (a) and (b)

(d) Contains cleavage site

17. M 13 is an example of

(a) Filamentous phage (b) Single stranded DNA vector

(c) Both (a) and (b) (d) Plasmid

18. Phagemid vectors are

(a) Combination of plasmid and phage λ

(b) Combination of phages and cosmid

(c) Phages carrying properties of plasmids

(d) All of the above

19. Single stranded vectors are useful

(a) For sequencing of cloned DNA

(b) For oligonucleotide directed mutagenesis

(c) For probe preparation

(d) All of the above

20. Inserted DNA in λ gt 11 can be expressed as

(a) β-galactosidase fused protein (b) Free protein in the cytoplasm

(c) Free protein that is secreted out (d) All of the above

21. EMBL 3 and EMBL 4 are replacement vectors, which can clone DNA up to

(a) 6-7 kb (b) 15-25 kb

(c) 40-44 kb (d) 1-2 kb

22. Size of the DNA that can be packaged into a λ phage is

(a) 50 kb (b) 35-53 kb

(c) 40-50 kb (d) Any size

23. Charon 34 and Charon 35 are the examples of

(a) Plasmid vector (b) Cosmid vector

(c) Phage vector (d) Phagemid vector

24. Cosmid vectors are used for

(a) Cloning small fragments of DNA (b) Cloning large fragments of DNA

(c) Cloning prokaryotic DNA only (d) Cloning eukaryotic DNA only

25. Plasmids which are maintained as limited number of copies per cell are known as

(a) Stringent plasmids (b) Relaxed plasmids

(c) Cryptic plasmids (d) All of these

26. Cryptic plasmids

(a) Do not exhibit any phenotypic trait (b) Exhibit one phenotypic traits

(c) Exhibit many phenotypic traits (d) Exhibit antibiotic resistance

27. Phagemid consist of

(a) Plasmid vector carrying λ phage's cos site

(b) Plasmid vector carrying λ attachment (λ att) site

(c) Plasmid vector carrying origin of replication of λ phage only

(d) Plasmid vector carrying origin of replication of plasmid only

28. Maximum size of foreign DNA that can be inserted into an insertion vector is

(a) 35 kb (b) 18 kb

(c) 50 kb (d) 27 kb

29. Plasmids which are maintained as multiple copy number per cell are known as

(a) Stringent plasmids (b) Relaxed plasmids

(c) Cryptic plasmids (d) None of these

30. Cosmid vectors are

(a) Plasmids that contain fragment of λ DNA including the cos site

(b) Phages that lack cos site

(c) Plasmids that have no selection marker

(d) Cryptic plasmids

31. Cosmids lack

(a) Genes coding for viral proteins

(b) Origin of replication

(c) Marker genes coding for replication

(d) Cleavage site for the insertion of foreign DNA

32. The monomers of DNA are bonded together to form _____.

(a) Polysaccharides (b) Polypeptides

(c) Polynucleotides (d) Polypentoses

33. _____ are subunits of DNA

(a) Amino acids (b) Nucleotides

(c) Monosaccharides (d) Fatty acids

34. A sugar containing five carbon atoms is a _____

(a) Triglyceride (b) Hexose
(c) Heptulose (d) Pentose

35. DNA contains a sugar component called _____.

(a) 1'-deoxyribose (b) 2'-deoxyribose
(c) 3'-deoxyribose (d) 4'-deoxyribose

36. A nucleoside does not contain a _____

(a) Pentose sugar (b) Nitrogenous base
(c) Phosphate group (d) Haworth structure

37. A 32-52 _____ bond serves as the linkage between monomers in DNA

(a) Ester (b) Phosphodiester
(c) Hydrogen (d) Ionic

38. One end of a polynucleotide has a(n) _____ terminus, and the other end has a(n) _____ terminus

(a) Amino group; 32-OH (b) Amino group, carboxyl group
(c) 5'-P; 3'-OH (d) Ester linkage; ester linkage

39. DNA directionality is _____

(a) 5' to 2' (b) 4' to 5'
(c) 5' to 3' (d) 3' to 2'

40. James Watson and Francis Crick reported that DNA is a _____

(a) Double helix (b) Beta-pleated sheet
(c) Alpha helix (d) Triple helix

41. Because the two polynucleotide polymers of DNA run in opposite orientation, they are _____

(a) Complementary (b) Asynchronous
(c) Antiparallel (d) Asymmetrical

42. DNA contains two grooves referred to as _____

(a) Large and small (b) Parallel and antiparallel
(c) A-form and B-form (d) Major and minor

43. The pairing between adjacent bases within the DNA helix utilizes _____

(a) Two purines or two pyrimidines (b) Ionic interactions
(c) Hydrogen bonds (d) Covalent bonds

44. Which of the following is not a permitted complementary base pair?

(a) Purine:pyrimidine
(b) T:A
(c) C:G
(d) Purine:purine

45. Watson and Crick based their analysis of DNA structure on the _____ of DNA

(a) B-form
(b) A-form
(c) C-form
(d) Z-form

46. Which of the following statements is incorrect regarding the different forms of the DNA double helix?

(a) Z-DNA is left-handed and assumes a zigzag conformation.
(b) B-DNA is the most tightly wound form with 12 bp per turn.
(c) A-DNA is more compact than B-DNA.
(d) B-DNA is the most common DNA in living cells.

47. A DNA sequence refers to the _____

(a) Rules pertaining to base pairing
(b) Linear order of nucleotides along a DNA strand
(c) Orientation of the base relative to the sugar
(d) Three-dimensional structure of a nucleotide

48. A polymer of DNA 20 nucleotides in length has _____ different sequence possibilities

(a) 20^4
(b) 20
(c) 4^{20}
(d) 10

49. _____ adds new nucleotides to the _____ end of the elongating strand during DNA replication.

(a) Polynucleotide phosphorylase; 32
(b) DNA polymerase: 32
(c) Replicase; 52
(d) Sequenase; 52

50. Template-dependent DNA synthesis makes sure that _____

(a) The product made retains the B-form
(b) Gene expression is always active
(c) The DNA strands are not antiparallel
(d) The double helix is an exact copy of the original pattern of nucleotides

51. The function of genes may be deduced from the _____

(a) Structure of the helix
(b) Sequence of nucleotides
(c) Base-pairing rules
(d) Contigs

52. **Long, uninterrupted stretches of DNA sequence making up _____ are determined by searching for overlaps of short DNA fragments**
    (a) Vectors (b) Primers
    (c) Contigs (d) Oligonucleotides

53. **Sonication is a method employing _____**
    (a) Enzymes to cleave DNA for cloning purposes
    (b) High frequency sound waves to fragment DNA
    (c) Computers to locate overlaps in DNA sequence
    (d) Chemicals to treat bacteria to facilitate uptake of recombinant vectors

54. **Cloning vectors are _____**
    (a) Exclusively linear DNA molecules
    (b) Able to replicate when introduced into Escherichia coli
    (c) Enzymes used to fragment DNA
    (d) Modified deoxynucleotides used for the chain termination method of DNA sequencing

55. **_____ is used to join together short DNA fragments and cloning vectors**
    (a) DNA ligase (b) DNA polymerase
    (c) DNA recombinase (d) DNA replicase

56. **A cloning vector that contains ligated DNA fragments is _____**
    (a) Competent (b) Recombinant
    (c) Primed (d) Polymerized

57. **A _____ is a collection of colonies containing recombinant vectors**
    (a) Competent assembly (b) Clone library
    (c) Contig (d) Oligonucleotide primer set

58. **When inserted into an elongating DNA strand _____ cause chain termination**
    (a) Dideoxynucleotides (b) Ribonucleotides
    (c) Deoxynucleotides (d) Trideoxynucleotides

59. **Separation of chain terminated fluorescent molecules during DNA sequencing uses a method called _____**
    (a) Agarose gel electrophoresis (b) Sonication
    (c) Restriction mapping (d) Capillary gel electrophoresis

Answers

1	(c)	16	(c)	31	(a)	46	(b)
2	(d)	17	(c)	32	(b)	47	(b)
3	(c)	18	(a)	33	(b)	48	(c)
4	(d)	19	(d)	34	(d)	49	(b)
5	(a)	20	(a)	35	(b)	50	(d)
6	(b)	21	(b)	36	(c)	51	(b)
7	(a)	22	(b)	37	(b)	52	(c)
8	(c)	23	(c)	38	(c)	53	(b)
9	(c)	24	(b)	39	(c)	54	(b)
10	(c)	25	(a)	40	(a)	55	(a)
11	(b)	26	(a)	41	(c)	56	(b)
12	(a)	27	(b)	42	(d)	57	(b)
13	(c)	28	(b)	43	(c)	58	(a)
14	(c)	29	(b)	44	(d)	59	(d)
15	(c)	30	(a)	45	(a)		

Chapter 25

Recombinant DNA

1. **The deliberate modifications of an organism's genetic information by directly changing its nucleic acid content is a subject matter of**
   - (a) Genetic engineering
   - (b) Population genetics
   - (c) Microbiology
   - (d) Protein engineering
2. **Enzymes that recognize and cleave specific 4 to 8 base pair sequences of DNA are**
   - (a) DNA ligase
   - (b) Helicases
   - (c) Restriction endonucleases
   - (d) DNA gyrase
3. **What is the normal role of restriction endonucleases in bacterial cells?**
   - (a) To degrade the bacterial chromosome into small pieces during replication
   - (b) To degrade invading phage DNA
   - (c) To produce RNA primers for replication
   - (d) All of the above
4. **Which type of restriction endonuclease cuts the DNA within the recognition site?**
   - (a) Type I
   - (b) Type II
   - (c) Type III
   - (d) All of the these
5. **Bacterial cells protect their own DNA from degradation by restriction endonucleases by**
   - (a) Methylating the DNA at the sites that the enzyme recognizes
   - (b) Deleting all recognition sites from the genome
   - (c) Not producing any restriction endonucleases
   - (d) Having anti restriction endonucleases

6. **Vectors are**
   (a) Molecules that degrade nucleic acids
   (b) Molecules that help in replication
   (c) Molecules that are able to covalently bond to and carry foreign DNA into cells
   (d) Molecules that protect host cells from invasion by foreign DNA

7. **Charged molecules are separated based on varying rates of migration through a solid matrix when subjected to an electric field. This technique is known as**
   (a) Photoreactivation (b) Gel electrophoresis
   (c) Autoradiography (d) Blotting

8. **The Southern blotting technique depends on**
   (a) Similarities between the sequences of probe DNA and experimental DNA
   (b) Similarities between the sequences of probe RNA and experimental RNA
   (c) Similarities between the sequences of probe protein and experimental protein
   (d) The molecular mass of proteins

9. **A short molecule containing 2-20 nucleotide is**
   (a) Plasmid (b) Vector
   (c) Oligonucleotide (d) Mononucleotide

10. **A molecular technique in which DNA sequences between two oligonucleotide primers can be amplified is known as**
   (a) Southern blotting (b) Northern blotting
   (c) Polymerase chain reaction (d) DNA replication

11. **The advantage of using DNA polymerases from thermophilic organisms in PCR is that**
   (a) The DNA polymerases of these bacteria are much faster than those from other organisms
   (b) The DNA polymerases of these bacteria can withstand the high temperatures needed to denature the DNA strands
   (c) The DNA polymerases of these bacteria never make mistakes while replicating DNA
   (d) All of the above

12. **Which of the following enzyme is used to covalently bond foreign DNA to a vector plasmid?**
   (a) DNA polymerase (b) Restriction endonuclease
   (c) DNA ligase (d) DNA helicase

13. A genomic library is

(a) A database where the sequence of an organism's genome is stored

(b) A collection of many clones possessing different DNA fragments from the same organisms bound to vectors

(c) A book that describes how to isolate DNA from a particular organism

(d) A place where the information of the genetic organization of organisms are kept

14. Which of the following is obtained using processed mRNA molecules as a template?

(a) *r*DNA (b) *m*DNA

(c) *c*DNA (d) *t*DNA

15. For gene probes to be useful they must

(a) Be large enough to contain gene-specific sequences

(b) Be labeled in some manner to allow detection

(c) Both (a) and (b)

(d) None of the above

16. Which of the following is not commonly used as vector?

(a) Artificial chromosome (b) Cosmid

(c) Fungi (d) Plasmid

17. In genetic engineering, a chimera is

(a) An enzyme that links DNA molecules

(b) A plasmid that contains foreign DNA

(c) A virus that infects bacteria

(d) A fungi

18. Which of the following vector can maintain the largest fragment of foreign DNA?

(a) YAC (b) Cosmid

(c) Plasmid (d) Phage

19. An animal, that has gained new genetic information from the acquisition of foreign DNA, is considered as

(a) An enzyme that links DNA molecules (b) A transgenic animal

(c) A vector (d) A chimera

20. Electroporation is

(a) The process of separating charged molecules through a gel maintained in an electric field

(b) The process of combining foreign DNA to an electrically charged vector molecule

(c) The application of high voltage pulses

(d) The process of multiplication of the cells

21. The piece of equipment, that introduces DNA into cells via DNA-coated micro projectiles is known as

(a) Laser | (d) Inoculating needle

(c) Gene gun | (b) DNA probe

22. Problems in obtaining large amounts of proteins encoded by recombinant genes can often be overcome by using

(a) BACS | (b) Expression vectors

(c) YACS | (d) All of these

23. Agrohacterium tutnefaciens is

(a) A disease in humans that causes loss of sight

(b) A bacterium that can be used to introduce DNA into plants

(c) A fungi that is used to produce antibiotics in large amounts

(d) A bacterium that can be used to introduce DNA into plants

Answers

1	(a)	7	(b)	13	(b)	19	(b)
2	(c)	8	(c)	14	(c)	20	(c)
3	(b)	9	(c)	15	(c)	21	(a)
4	(b)	10	(c)	16	(c)	22	(d)
5	(a)	11	(b)	17	(c)	23	(b)
6	(c)	12	(c)	18	(a)		

Chapter 26

Recombinant DNA Technology for the Synthesis of Therapeutic Agents

1. **The first therapeutic product formed by means of recombinant DNA technology is**
   (a) Vaccine for foot and mouth disease
   (b) Insulin
   (c) Hepatitis B vaccine
   (d) Human growth hormone

2. **Human insulin formed by recombinant DNA technology is known as**
   (a) H insulin
   (b) R insulin
   (c) Humulin
   (d) Huinsulin

3. **How is human insulin synthesized using recombinant DNA technology?**
   (a) By using chemically synthesized DNA sequences for the two chains separately
   (b) By isolating DNA from the islets of Langerhans of pancreas
   (c) By using cDNA for insulin
   (d) By using chemically synthesized DNA sequences for the complete insulin protein

4. **Chemically synthesized DNA sequences for the two chains are separately inserted into the plasmid pBR 322 by the side of**
   (a) β-Galactosidase
   (b) Galactokinase
   (c) Acid phosphatase
   (d) Glucokinase

5. **The two chains of insulin can be separated by detaching it from β-galactosidase using**
   (a) Hydrogen chloride
   (b) Cyanogen bromide
   (c) Peptidase
   (d) Protease

6. **The two chains are joined together to constitute native insulin using**
   (a) Sodium dissulphonate and sodium sulphite
   (b) Sodium dissulphonate and sodium sulphate
   (c) Sodium sulphate and sodium sulphite
   (d) Sodium sulphate only

7. **Human growth hormone (hGH) is secreted by**
   (a) Pitutary gland (b) Hypothalamus
   (c) Pancreas (d) None of these

8. **The recombinant hGH lacks**
   (a) Terminal glutamine (b) Terminal lysine
   (c) Terminal methionine (d) Terminal arginine

9. **Recombinant vaccine for Hepatitis B virus has been synthesized against which of the following antigen?**
   (a) Viral core antigen (HBcAg) (b) Viral surface antigen (HBcAg)
   (c) E antigen (HBeAg) (d) All of the above

10. **Recombinant vaccine for HBV was produced by cloning viral genes in**
    (a) Plasmids
    (b) Cosmids
    (c) Autonomously replicating plasmid of yeast
    (d) Phagemids

11. **The promoter used for cloning HBV surface antigen is**
    (a) Galactokinase (b) Alcohol dehydrogenase I
    (c) β-galactosidase (d) Polyhedrin

12. **In India first genetically engineered vaccine against HBV was developed by**
    (a) Ranbaxy Pvt Ltd (b) Shantha Biotechnics Pvt Ltd
    (c) Dabur Pvt Ltd (d) Glaxo Pvt Ltd

13. **Foot and mouth disease (FMD) of animals is caused by**
    (a) RNA virus (b) DNA virus
    (c) Bacteria (d) Protozoa

14. **How many nucleotides are there in Ss RNA molecule of picorna virus causing FMD?**
    (a) 1000 (b) 5000
    (c) 8000 (d) 10000

15. Which one of the following capsid protein of picorna virus is immunogenic in nature?

(a) VP1 (b) VP2

(c) VP3 (d) VP4

16. The gene coding for VPI is cloned in

(a) PMB 9 (b) PBR 322

(c) PUC 18 (d) PUC 19

Answers

1	(b)	5	(b)	9	(b)	13	(a)
2	(c)	6	(a)	10	(c)	14	(c)
3	(a)	7	(a)	11	(b)	15	(a)
4	(a)	8	(c)	12	(b)	16	(b)

Chapter 27
Tissue Culture

1. **Who is the father of tissue culture?**
   (a) Bonner (b) Haberlandt
   (c) Laibach (d) Gautheret
2. **The production of secondary metabolites require the use of**
   (a) Protoplast (b) Cell suspension
   (c) Meristem (d) Auxillary buds
3. **Synthetic seed is produced by encapsulating somatic embryo with**
   (a) Sodium chloride (b) Sodium alginate
   (c) Sodium acetate (d) Sodium nitrate
4. **Hormone pair required for a callus to differentiate are**
   (a) Auxin and cytokinin (b) Auxin and ethylene
   (c) Auxin and absiccic acid (d) Cytokinins and gibberllin
5. **DMSO (Dimethyl sulfoxide) is used as**
   (a) Gelling agent (b) Alkaylating agent
   (c) Chelating agent (d) Cryoprotectant
6. **The most widely used chemical for protoplast fusion, as fusogens, is**
   (a) Manitol (b) Sorbitol
   (c) Mannol (d) Poly ethylene glycol (PEG)
7. **Cybridsare produced by**
   (a) Fusion of two different nuclei from two different species
   (b) Fusion of two same nuclei from same species
   (c) Nucleus of one species but cytoplasm from both the parent species
   (d) None of the above

8. **Callus is**
   (a) Tissue that forms embryo
   (b) An insoluble carbohydrate
   (c) Tissue that grows to form embryoid
   (d) Un organised actively dividing mass of cells maintained in cultured

9. **Part of plant used for culturing is called**
   (a) Scion (b) Explant
   (c) Stock (d) Callus

10. **Growth hormone producing apical dominance is**
   (a) Auxin (b) Gibberellin
   (c) Ethylene (d) Cytokinin

11. **A medium which is composed of chemically defined compound is called**
   (a) Natural media (b) Synthetic media
   (c) Artificial media (d) None of these

12. **To obtain haploid plant, we culture**
   (a) Entire anther (b) Nucleus
   (c) Embryo (d) Apical bud

13. **Somaclonal variations are the ones**
   (a) Caused by mutagens (b) Produce during tissue culture
   (c) Induced during sexual embryogeny (d) Caused by gamma rays

14. **Which of the following plant cell will show totipotency?**
   (a) Xylem vessels (b) Sieve tube
   (c) Meristem (d) Cork cells

15. **Which vector is mostly used in crop improvement?**
   (a) Plasmid (b) Cosmid
   (c) Phasmid (d) Agrobacterium

Answers

1	(b)	5	(d)	9	(b)	13	(b)
2	(b)	6	(d)	10	(a)	14	(c)
3	(b)	7	(c)	11	(b)	15	(d)

Chapter 28
Plant Tissue Culture Techniques

1. **The tumor phenotype, which can be maintained indefinitely in tissue culture, results from the expression of genes on the**
   (a) T-DNA (b) cDNA
   (c) r-DNA (d) m-RNA
2. **Which of the following have been used for cryo-preservation of germplasm with 90 per cent tissue survival and 10 per cent plant regeneration that are used in international exchange of germplasm?**
   (a) Meristem culture
   (b) Embryo culture
   (c) Both (a) and (b)
   (d) Embryo cultures supplemented with GA_3 and coconut milk
3. **Establishment of embryogenic cell suspensions with high regeneration potential is a pre-requisite for successful**
   (a) Protoplast culture
   (b) Detection of nucleic acid sequence
   (c) Restriction of fragment length polymorphisms
   (d) Mircoinjection
4. **The tumor phenotype, which can be maintained indefinitely in tissue culture, results from the expression of genes on the**
   (a) T-DNA (b) c-DNA
   (c) r-DNA (d) m-RNA
5. **Which of the following have been used for cryo-preservation of germplasm with 90 per cent tissue survival and 10 per cent plant regeneration that are used in international exchange of germplasm?**
   (a) Meristem tip cultures (b) Embryo cultures
   (c) Embryo cultures supplemented with GA_3 and coconut milk (d) Both (a) and (b)

6. **Establishment of embryogenic cell suspensions with high regeneration potential is a pre-requisite for successful**
   (a) Protoplast culture
   (b) detection of nucleic acid sequence
   (c) Restriction of fragment length polymorphisms
   (d) Microinjection

7. **Which of the following technique can be used to develop nematode resistant plants?**
   (a) Embryo-rescue (b) Mutation
   (c) Non-recombinant DNA (d) All of these

8. **Random amplified polymorphic DNA (RAPD) is a method that**
   (a) Stimulate production of sense RNA to compensate
   (b) Activate the expression of all genes in a biochemical pathway
   (c) Eliminate the expression of all genes in a biochemical pathway
   (d) Reveals intra-specific variation and diversity between species

9. **Which of the following transfers a set of genes encoded in a region called T-DNA of the Ti-plasmid into cells at wound positions?**
   (a) *A. tumefaciens* (b) *L. peruvianum*
   (c) *L. birsutum* (d) *A. sterilis*

10. **Which of the following govern sporophytic self-incompatibility in *Brassica*?**
   (a) Aegilops (b) Triticum
   (c) Both (a) and (b) (d) S alleles

11. **Commercial sugarcane is heterozygons with germplasm from**
   (a) 1-3 *Saccharum* species (b) 3-5 *Saccharum* species
   (c) 5-7 *Saccharum* species (d) 7-9 *Saccharum* species

12. **The intervention in the communication system of nematodes offer several possibilities of bio control. Which of the following(s) play(s) a very important role in the host recognition?**
   (a) Protein (b) Lipid
   (c) Carbohydrate moiety (d) Minerals

13. **The hybrid embryo can be rescued from damage/collapse by growing it**
   (a) At low temperature (b) At low pH
   (c) At low water activity (d) In artificial medium

14. For increased level of mannitol in transgenic tobacco plants which of the following gene is transferred?

(a) Mannitol dehydrogenase (b) Mannitol synthease

(c) Both (a) and (b) (d) Mannitol pyrophosphorylase

15. Meristem culture of banana enables

(a) Elimination of bunch top virus disease (b) Rapid multiplication

(c) Both (a) and (b) (d) Slow growth

16. Wheat variety Rendezvous, with resistance to eye spot (*Pseudo-cercosporella herpotrichoides*) derived from *Aegilops ventricosa*, has a chloroplast genome derived from

(a) Aegilops (b) Triticum

(c) Both (a) and (b) (d) S alleles

17. Human serum albumin in case of transgenic plant is secreted in

(a) Transgenic leaf tissues (b) Transgenic root tissues

(c) Is not secreted out of plant (d) Transgenic stem tissues

18. Protoplast fusion technique generally involves

(a) Hybridization between two species (b) Isolation and fusion

(c) Isolation, fusion and culturing (D) Isolation only

19. Cytoplast (somatic cell hybridization) is the process in which

(a) Two protoplast along with their nuclei fuse

(b) A normal protoplast along with an enucleated protoplast fuse

(c) Both (a) and (b)

(d) Two enucleated protoplasts fuse

20. Somaclonal variation method refers to

(a) Heritable changes

(b) Genetic isolation

(c) Small number of species having limited commercial potential

(d) Large number of plant cells

21. α and β cyclo dextrins are produced by

(a) Transgenic tomato (b) Transgenic maize

(c) Transgenic potato (d) Transgenic wheat

22. α and β cyclo dextrins are used for

(a) Pharmaceutical delivery system

(b) Flavour and odour enhancement in foods

(c) Removal of undesired compounds like caffeine from foods
(d) All of the above

23. Microinjection technique of introducing NA is a
(a) Physical method
(b) Biological method
(b) Combination of physical and biological method
(d) Chemical method

24. MS medium, is found essential for initial morphogenesis of the immature embryos and to enhance callus development, when supplemented with
(a) GA_3
(b) GA_3 and coconut milk
(c) Adenine
(d) Adenine and kinetin

25. Plant tissue culture technique is used to select somaclones that are
(a) Resistant to herbicide
(b) Not resistant to herbicide
(c) Resistant to insecticides
(d) Not resistant to insecticides

26. Which of the following mutant/(s) has/have increased amount of lysine and/ or methionine in corn seeds?
(a) Opaque-2
(b) Sugary-1
(c) Flory-2
(d) All of these

27. Which of the following is the class of hybridization?
(a) Intervarietal
(b) Interspecific
(c) Intergeneric
(d) All of these

28. Cultivated tomato species (*Lycopersicon esculentum*) is highly susceptible to
(a) *Meloidogyne* spp. nematodes
(b) *L. peruviaanum*
(c) Both (a) and (b)
(d) *Solarium melongena*

29. In transgenic plants of *Arabidipsis thaliana* which of the following gene is transferred for the synthesis of PHB (polyhdroxybutyrate)?
(a) Polyhydroxybutyrate synthease
(b) Acetyl Co A reductase
(c) Both (a) and (b)
(d) Pyrophosphorylase

30. Cultivated tomato species (*Lycopersicon esculentum*) has a high degree of resistance towards
(a) *Meloidogyne* spp. nematodes
(b) *L. peruviaanum*
(b) Both (a) and (b)
(d) *Solarium melongena*

31. When the transposon jumps into an otherwise functional gene, it has the effect of

(a) Blocking correct transcription
(b) Initiating correct transcription
(b) Propagating correct transcription
(d) Initiating some genetic codes

32. cDNA clone prepared to stigma mRNA of *Brassica oleracea* can be used as a probe on DNA digests of segregating populations to recognize

(a) Aegilops
(b) Triticum
(c) Both (a) and (b)
(d) S alleles

33. Virulence trait of *Agrobacterium tumefaciens* is borne on

(a) Tumour inducing plasmid DNA
(b) Chromosomal DNA
(c) Both chromosomal and plasmid DNA
(d) Cryptic plasmid DNA

34. The size of the virulent plasmid of *Agrobacterium tumefaciens* is

(a) 40-80 kb
(b) 80-120 kb
(c) 140-235 kb
(d) >235 kb

35. Which of the following is not true about the helper plasmids?

(a) These can replicate in *Agrobacterium*
(b) These help in the mediating conjugation of intermediate vectors
(c) These can't replicate in *Agrobacterium*
(d) All of the above

36. Which technique is used to introduce genes into dicots?

(a) Electroporation
(b) particle acceleration
(c) Microinjection
(d) Ti plasmid infection

37. Direct DNA uptake by protoplasts can be stimulated by

(a) Polyethylene glycol (PEG)
(b) Decanal
(c) Luciferin
(d) All of these

38. In a plant tumour cell

(a) Complete Ti plasmid is incorporated in plant nuclear DNA
(b) Different parts of the Ti-plasmid are incorporated
(c) Only a small specific segment of callus T DNA is incorporated
(d) May vary from plant to plant

39. Co-integrating transformation vectors must include a region of homology in

(a) The vector plasmid
(b) The Ti-plasmid
(c) Between vector plasmid and Ti-plasmid
(d) None of these

40. Crown gall tissue

(a) Can be cultivated in vitro in absence of bacteria

(b) Retains tumorous properties when cultivated

(c) Both (a) and (b)

(d) Shows tumorous properties only in presence of bacteria

41. Integrated nopaline T-DNA occurs as

(a) Single segment (b) Two segments

(c) Three segments (d) Four segments

42. Which of the following is true about *Agrobacterium tumefaciens*?

(a) It causes crown gall disease of plants (b) It infects gymosperms

(c) It infects dicotyledonous angiosperms (d) All of the above

43. In the liposome mediated gene transfer in plants, nucleic acids are

(a) Protected from nuclease digestion (b) Stable in liposomes

(c) Both (a) and (b) (d) Not stable in liposomes

44. Advantage of microprojectile method over microinjection method for gene transfer in plants include

(a) Intact cells are used

(b) Method is universal in its application irrespective of all shape, size, type and presence or absence of cell wall

(c) Gene can be transferred to many cells simultaneously

(d) All of the above

45. On Ti-plasmid T-region or T-DNA is flanked by a direct repeat of

(a) 12 bp (b) 20 bp

(c) 25 bp (d) 30 bp

46. *Agrobacterium tumefaciens* is a

(a) Gram (+) bacteria (b) Gram (–) bacteria

(c) A fungi (d) A yeast

47. Microprojectile method of gene transfer in plants involves delivery of DNA

(a) With the help of micromanipulator (b) With the help of bolistics

(c) With the help of needles (d) Any of the above

48. Which of the following genes are constitutively expressed and control the plant induced activation of other vir genes?

(a) *Vir* A and *vir* G (b) *Vir* C and *vir* D

(c) *Vir* B and *vir* E (d) *Vir* A and *vir* B

49. Liposomes mediated gene transfer in plants involves

(a) Plasmid DNA enclosed in a lipid bag

(b) Fusion of liposomes with protoplast

(c) Use of polyethylene glycol (PEG)

(d) All of the above

50. Which of the following plant signal molecules regulate the expression of vir B, C, D and E in case of tobacco?

(a) Acetosyringone (b) α-hydroxy syringone

(c) Both (a) and (b) (d) None of these

51. Opines that are present in crown gall tumour include

(a) Octopine (b) Nopaline

(c) Agropine (d) All of these

52. Intermediate vectors containing T-DNA are conjugation deficient. Thus conjugation is mediated in presence of which of the following plasmid?

(a) PRK 2013 (b) pRN 3

(c) Either (a) or (b) (d) None of these

53. Which of the following is true about T DNA?

(a) Integration of T DNA can occur at many different, apparently random, sites in the plant nuclear DNA

(b) Integration of T DNA occurs only at one specific sites in the plant nuclear DNA

(c) Integration of T DNA occurs at two specific sites in the plant nuclear DNA

(d) Integration of T DNA occurs at one site that may be random in the plant nuclear DNA

54. Which of the following is not true about the direct repeats flanking T-DNA?

(a) They are conserved between nopaline and octopine Ti-plasmids

(b) These repeats are transferred intact to the plant genome

(c) These are important in integration mechanism

(d) All of the above

55. The left segment of octopine T-DNA (TL) is necessary for

(a) Enzymes for agropine biosynthesis (b) Tumour formation

(c) Conjugative transfer (d) All of these

56. Which of the following is not true for microinjection technique that involves transfer of DNA into protoplast?

(a) It is carried out with the help of micromanipulator

(b) The recipient cells are immobilized on artificial support or artificially bound to substarate
(c) It employs needle with diameter greater than cell diameter
(d) All of the above

57. The right segment of octopine T-DNA (TR) is necessary for
(a) Enzymes for agropine biosynthesis
(b) Tumour formation
(c) Conjugative transfer
(d) All of these

58. Opine synthesis is the property
(a) Conferred to plant cells when it transformed by *Agrobacterium tumefaciens*
(b) Determined by the bacteria *Agrobacterium tumefaciens*
(c) Both (a) and (b)
(d) Of normal plant cells

59. Virulent strains of Agrobacterium contain large Ti-plasmids, which are responsible for the DNA transfer and subsequent disease symptoms. It has been shown that Ti-plasmids contain
(a) One set of sequence necessary for gene transfer
(b) Two sets of sequence necessary for gene transfer
(c) Three sets of sequence necessary for gene transfer
(d) Four sets of sequence necessary for gene transfer

60. The direct repeats flanking the T-DNA of *Agrobacterium tume-faciens* are known as
(a) Cos site
(b) Flanking sequences
(c) Border sequences
(d) Transfer sequences

61. T-DNA transfer and processing into plant genome requires products of which of the following genes?
(a) *Vir* A,B
(b) *Vir* G,C
(c) *Vir* D,E
(d) All of these

62. Because of large size of Ti-plasmid, intermediate vectors (IV) are developed in which T DNA has been subcloned into
(a) PBR 322 based plasmid vector
(b) pRK 2013
(c) pRN 3
(d) All of these

63. The transfer of intermediate vectors into *Agrobacterium* are brought about by
(a) Transformation
(b) Biparental mating
(c) Triparental mating
(d) Transduction

64. In response to the activating signal molecule, an endonuclease is produced that causes nicks in the T-DNA. It is encoded by

(a) *Vir* A (b) *Vir* B

(c) *Vir* C (d) *Vir* D

65. Microinjection involves

(a) Injection of large amount of DNA

(b) Injection of DNA into bigger cells

(c) Injection with needle having diameter greater than cell diameter

(d) All of the above

66. Which of the following are used as selection marker for the cells transformed with*Agrobacterium*?

(a) Neomycin phosphotransferase

(b) Streptomycin phosphotransferase

(b) Hygromycin phosphotransferase

(d) Any of the above

67. Vir genes required for the T-DNA transfer and processing are located

(a) On the T-DNA (b) Outside the T-DNA region

(c) On the plant genome (d) None of these

68. Plant transformation vectors based on *Agrobacterium* can generally be divided into

(a) Two vectors (b) Four vectors

(c) Six vectors (d) Eight vectors

69. Which of the following plant signal molecules regulate the expression of vir B, C, D and E in case of tobacco?

(a) Acetosyringone (b) α-hydroxy syringone

(c) Both (a) and (b) (d) None of these

70. Synthetic seeds are

(a) Artificially synthesized seeds

(b) Somatic embryos encapsulated in suitable matrix

(c) Seeds of plants modified genetically

(d) Bone of these

71. Somatic embryoids are

(a) Identical with zygotic embryos and without seed coats

(b) Identical with zygotic embryos and with seed coats

(c) Non-identical with zygotic embryos and without seed coats
(d) Non-identical with zygotic embryos and with seed coats

72. The production of high quality and uniform embryos has been limited to only
(a) Carrot (b) Alfalfa
(c) Both (a) and (b) (d) Sandalwood

73. The preserved embryoids are termed as
(a) Synthetic seeds (b) Semi-synthetic seeds
(c) Natural seeds (d) Fermented seeds

74. Encapsulation is necessary to produce and protect synthetic seeds. The encapsulation is carried out by various types of hydrogels, which are
(a) Soluble in water (b) Soluble in organic solvents
(c) Insoluble in water (d) Insoluble in organic solvents

75. Which of the following is not true about synthetic seeds?
(a) Can be stored for a year without the loss of valuables
(b) Easy to handle
(c) Can be directly sown in the soil like natural seeds
(d) Need hardening in the green house

76. Recalcitrant seeds are
(a) Resistant to drying and freezing temperature
(b) Killed by drying and freezing temperature
(c) Both (a) and (b)
(d) None of above

77. The encapsulation of somatic embryos can be carried out by
(a) Automatic encapsulation process (b) Gel complexation
(c) Both (a) and (b) (d) Coating proteins

78. The yield of the antibiotic depends upon
(a) pH of the medium (b) Age of the inoculum
(c) Composition of the medium (d) All of these

79. During which phase of growth of *Penicillium chrysogenum* maximum antibiotic production takes place
(a) During the first phase (b) During the second phase
(c) During the third phase (d) Same in all the phases

80. Fermentation medium for oxytetracyclin (terramycin) consist of

(a) CSL, starch, $(NH_4)_2 SO_4$, sodium chloride and $CaCO_3$

(b) CSL, $(NH_4)_2 SO_4$, sodium chloride and $CaCO_3$

(c) CSL, starch, $(NH_4)_2 SO_4$, ammonium chloride and $CaCO_3$

(d) CSL, $(NH_4)_2 SO_4$, ammonium chloride and $CaCO_3$

81. pH of the fermentation medium for chlorotetracyclins is

(a) 5-6 (b) 6-7

(c) 7-8 (d) 8-9

82. At normal pH, penicillin remains in

(a) Aqueous phase (b) Solvent phase

(c) Both (a) and (b) (d) Precipitates

83. At acidic pH, penicillin remains in

(a) Aqueous phase (b) Solvent phase

(c) Both (a) and (b) (d) Precipitates

84. Chlorotetracyclin is soluble in

(a) Organic solvents (b) Water

(c) Either (d) All of these

85. Penicillin is produced by

(a) Aerobic fermentation

(b) anaerobic fermentation

(c) Aerobic fermentation followed by anaerobic fermentation

(d) Anaerobic fermentation followed by aerobic fermentation

86. Penicillin is recovered after fermentation as

(a) Potassium penicillin (b) Calcium penicillin

(c) Sodium penicillin (d) Penicillin only

87. Media composition for the production of streptomycin is

(a) Soybean meal, glucose, peptone, malt extract, sodium chloride

(b) Soybean meal, glucose, peptone, malt extract, ammonium chloride

(c) Soybean meal, glucose, peptone, malt extract, calcium carbonate

(d) Soybean meal, glucose, peptone, malt extract, ammonium sulphate

88. Which of the following organism(s) produce(s) tetracycline?

(a) *Steptomyces aureofaciens* (b) *Steptomyces ramosus*

(c) *Nocardia sulphurea* (d) All of these

89. Media used for the production of chlorotetracyclin consists of

(a) Sugar, corn steep liquor, $CaCO_3$, $(NH_4)_2SO_4$ and NH_4Cl

(b) Corn steep liquor, $CaCO_3$ and $(NH_4)_2SO_4$

(c) Sugar, $CaCO_3$ and $(NH_4)_2SO_4$

(d) Corn steep liquor, $CaCO_3$, $(NH_4)_2SO_4$ and NH_4Cl

90. Which of the following precursor is added in the medium to get penicillin G?

(a) Phenyl carbamic acid (b) Phenyl acetic acid

(c) Ammonium sulphate (d) Ammonium chloride

91. High yield of chlorotetracyclin requires

(a) No aeration (b) Continuous aeration

(c) Aeration which does not affect the yield (d) Controlled aeration

92. Streptomycin is produced by

(a) *S. griseus* (b) *S. griseoflavus*

(c) *S. aerofaciens* (d) *S. ramosus*

93. Which of the following event occurs during second phase of growth of *P. chrysogenum*?

(a) Synthesis of penicillin is high (b) Mycelial mass increases

(c) pH increase (d) Both (a) and (b)

94. Inoculum preparation for the fermentation medium for penicillin takes place on

(a) Wheat seeds (b) Barley seeds

(c) Rice seeds (d) All of these

95. Antibiotics are typically produced in fed batch reactors because

(a) Antibiotic yields are generally higher when cells enter the stationary phase

(b) The precursors are often toxic to the cells

(c) Antibiotic yields are generally higher when cell growth slows

(d) All of the above

96. Which of the following event occurs during third phase of growth of *P. chrysogenum*?

(a) Concentration of antibiotic increases in the medium

(b) Autolysis of the medium starts

(c) Slight rise in pH due to liberation of ammonia

(d) All of the above

97. Vegetable oil, (corn oil or soybean oil) added in the fermentation medium for penicillin, act as

(a) Source of nutrients
(b) Carbon source
(c) Antifoam agent
(d) Both (a) and (c)

98. Which of the following changes occur during first phase of growth of *Penicillium chrysogenum*?

(a) Growth of mycelia occurs
(b) Ammonia is liberated in the medium
(c) Lactic acid present in the corn steep liquor is utilized at the maximum rate
(d) All of the above

99. The most common carbon source used in the plant cell culture media?

(a) Sucrose
(b) Glucose
(c) Fructose
(d) Maltose

100. Which of the following is an ethylene biosynthesis inhibitor?

(a) Citric acid
(b) Succinic acid
(c) Activated charcoal
(d) Silver thiosulphate

101. Nitrogen in the plant cell culture media is provided by either ammonia or nitrate salt. In the media

(a) Utilization of ammonium cause culture pH to drop while utilization of nitrate cause culture pH to rise
(b) Utilization of nitrate cause culture pH to drop while utilization of ammonium cause culture pH to rise
(c) Utilization of both ammonium and nitrate result in rise in pH
(d) Utilization of both ammonium and nitrate result in drop in pH

102. Which of the following growth regulator is added for short initiation during plant regeneration from callus?

(a) Auxins
(b) Cytokinins
(c) Gibberellins
(d) Brassinosteroids

103. Which of the following growth regulator promote cell division?

(a) Auxins
(b) Cytokinins
(c) Gibberellins
(d) Brassinosteroids
(a) Auxins B. Cytokinins C. Gibberellins D. Brassinosteroids

104. Which of the following growth regulator is used to stimulate embryo or shoot development?

(a) Auxins
(b) Cytokinins
(c) Gibberellins
(d) Brassinosteroids

105. Which of the following growth regulator cause plant cells to grow?

(a) Auxins (b) Cytokinins

(c) Gibberellins (d) Brassinosteroids

106. Silver thiosulphate is added to culture medium as it helps to

(a) Maintain the pH

(b) Remove toxic phenolics from plant cells

(c) Prevent the gaseous plant hormone, ethylene dioxide from accumulating to detrimental condition.

(d) All of the above

107. In plant cell culture media, auxins and cytokinins are used in the range of

(a) 1-50µM (b) 50-100µM

(c) 100-125µM (d) more than 125µM

108. Concentration of sucrose generally used in plant cell culture media is

(a) 10-15 g/l (b) 20-30 g/l

(c) 40-50 g/l (d) 60-70 g/l

109. Which is/are the naturally occurring plant auxins?

(a) Indole acetic acid (IAA)

(b) Naphthalenacetic acid (NAA)

(c) 2,4-dichlorophenoxyacetic acid

(d) All of the above

110. Which is/are the disadvantage/(s) of using IAA in plant cell culture media?

(a) It is unstable in solution

(b) Gets easily oxidized

(c) Conjugated to inactive form by plant cells

(d) All of the above

111. To maintain the pH of the culture

(a) Organic acid such as citric, fumaric, malic and succinic acid is used

(b) Synthetic buffers such as Tris, MES or HEPS are used

(c) Both (a) and (b)

(d) Ammonium salts are used

112. Which of the following is not a cytokinin?

(a) 2,4-dichlorophenoxyacetic acid (b) 6-benzylaminopurine

(c) Zeatin (d) Kinetin

113. Which of the following is not an auxin?

(a) Naphthalenacetic acid (NAA)
(b) Indole acetic acid (IAA)
(c) Zeatin
(d) Indole butyric acid

114. Which of the following is not true about nurse or conditioned medium?

(a) It is liquid removed from the suspension of fast growing cells
(b) It contains uncharacterized growth factor released by growing cells
(c) It is used in the culture of regenerating protoplast
(d) It is removed aseptically from the culture and is autoclaved before use

115. Very high sugar concentration (40-100 g/l) have been used

(a) In specialized secondary metabolite production
(b) To adjust the osmotic potential of the media in short term treatment for regeneration
(c) Both (a) and (b)
(d) None of these

116. What is 'nurse' or conditioned medium?

(a) It is the media full of growth factors used for the growth of cells
(b) It is the medium added to nurse the callus culture
(c) Both (a) and (b)
(d) It is the liquid medium removed from the suspension of fast growing cells

117. What are the macronutrients used in plant cell culture medium?

(a) N, P, K, S, Na
(b) N, P, K, Ca, Cl
(c) N, P, K, S, Ca
(d) N, P, Ca, Na, Cl

118. Neutralized activated charcoal is occasionally added to young regenerating cultures to

(a) Remove toxic phenolics produced by the stressed plant cell
(b) Help to remove plants growth regulators introduced at an earlier stage
(c) Both (a) and (b)
(d) Maintain the pH of the medium

119. A(*n*) __________ is an excised piece of leaf or stem tissue used in micropropagation.

(a) Microshoot
(b) Medium
(c) Extant
(d) Scion

120. Protoplasts can be produced from suspension cultures, callus tissues or intact tissues by enzymatic treatment with

(a) Cellulotyic enzymes

(b) Pectolytic enzymes

(c) Both cellulotyic and pectolytic enzymes

(d) Proteolytic enzymes

121. Which of the following is considered as the disadvantage of conventional plant tissue culture for clonal propagation?

(a) Multiplication of sexually derived sterile hybrids

(b) Less multiplication of disease free plants

(c) Storage and transportation of propogates

(d) Both (b) and (c)

122. What is meant by 'Organ culture' ?

(a) Maintenance alive of a whole organ, after removal from the organism by partial immersion in a nutrient fluid

(b) Introduction of a new organ in an animal body with a view to create genetic mutation in the progenies of that animal

(c) Cultivation of organs in a laboratory through the synthesis of tissues

(d) The aspects of culture in community which are mainly dedicated by the need of a specified organ of the human body

123. Which method of plant propagation involves the use of girdling?

(a) Grafting (b) Cuttings

(c) Layering (d) Micropropagation

124. Organogenesis is

(a) Formation of callus tissue

(b) Formation of root and shoots on callus tissue

(c) Both (a) and (b)

(d) Genesis of organs

125. Which of the following is used in the culture of regenerating protoplasts, single cells or very dilute cell suspensions?

(a) Nurse medium (b) Nurse or feeder culture

(c) Both (a) and (b) (d) None of these

126. In a callus culture

(a) Increasing level of cytokinin to a callus induces shoot formation and increasing level of auxin promote root formation

(b) Increasing level of auxin to a callus induces shoot formation and increasing level of cytokinin promote root formation

(c) Auxins and cytokinins are not required
(d) Only auxin is required for root and shoot formation

127. Protoplasts are the cells devoid of

(a) Cell membrane (b) Cell wall
(c) Both cell wall and cell membrane (d) None of these

128. Which breeding method uses a chemical to strip the cell wall of plant cells of two sexually incompatible species?

(a) Mass selection (b) Protoplast fusion
(c) Transformation (d) Transpiration

129. The phenomenon of the reversion of mature cells to the meristematic state leading to the formation of callus is known as

(a) Redifferentiation (b) Dedifferentiation
(c) Either (a) or (b) (d) None of these

130. Cell fusion method includes the preparation of large number of

(a) Plant cells stripped of their cell wall
(b) Single plant cell stripped of their cell wall
(c) Plant cells with cell wall
(d) Cells from different species

131. Subculturing is similar to propagation by cuttings because

(a) It separates multiple microshoots and places them in a medium
(b) It uses scions to produce new microshoots
(c) They both use in vitro growing conditions
(d) All of the above

132. The ability of the component cells of callus to form a whole plant is known as

(a) Redifferentiation (b) Dedifferentiation
(c) Either (a) or (b) (d) None of these

133. What is/are the benefit(s) of micropropagation or clonal propagation?

(a) Rapid multiplication of superior clones
(b) Multiplication of disease free plants
(c) Multiplication of sexually derived sterile hybrids
(d) All of the above

134. When plated only in nutrient medium, how much time is required for the protoplast to synthesize new cell wall?

(a) 2-5 days (b) 5-10 days
(c) 10-15 days (d) 15-17 days

135. Cellular totipotency is the property of

(a) Plants (b) Animals

(c) Bacteria (d) All of these

136. Agrobacterium based gene transfer is efficient

(a) Only with dicots

(b) Only with monocots

(c) with both monocots and dicots

(d) With majority monocots and few dicots

137. Genetic potential to reproduce the entire organism

(a) Pluropotent (b) Totipotent

(c) Both (a) and (b) (d) None of these

138. The most important commercial technique for micropropagating plants is known as

(a) Shoot-tip culture (b) Meristem culture

(c) Tissue culture (d) Organ culture

139. Plants with gametic chromosome number are termed as which of the following

(a) Diploid (b) Dihaploid

(c) Haploid (d) Monoploid

140. During distant hybridization, problem of endosperm abortion can be overcome by which of following?

(a) Embryo culture (b) Ovary culture

(c) Ovule culture (d) All the above

141. Sometic embryos can be used for which of the following?

(a) Genetic transformation

(b) Production of uniform plant population

(c) *In vitro* mutagenesis

(d) All of the above

142. Somaclonal variation occurs due to which of the following?

(a) Methylation and demethylation in the promoter region of gene

(b) Activation of silent genes in multigene family

(c) Non-reciprocal mitotic recombination

(d) All of the above

143. Guha and maheswari produced haploids from anther cultures of which of the following:

(a) Nicotiana (b) Datura

(c) Ginkgo (d) Hordeum

144. Somaclonal variation generally serves the purpose as which of the following?

(a) Analytical breeding (b) Mutation breeding

(c) Back cross breeding (d) Hybrid sorting

145. Cryopreservation is based on which of the following?

(a) Liquid CO_2 (b) Liquid helium

(c) Liquid nitrogen (d) Both (a) and (b)

146. Which of the following scientist is regarded as father of plant tissue culture?

(a) Herbert E. Street (b) Gottlieb Haberlandt

(c) Jean P. Nitsch (d) Phillip R. White

147. The term somaclonal variation was coined by which of the following scientists?

(a) Vasil and vasil (b) Lakrin and Scow croft

(c) Skirvin and Karp (d) Evans and Sharp

148. Pusa Jaikisan (Bio 902) Somaclone of Indian mustard was isolated from which of following varieties?

(a) Pusa bold (b) Kranti

(c) Varuna (d) Karuna

149. During Gynogenesis, haploid plants generally originate from which of the following?

(a) Synergids (b) Antipodal cells

(c) Egg cell (d) Polar nuclei

150. Anther culture ordinarily yield which of the following

(a) Haploid plants (b) Disomic plants

(c) Polyploid plant (d) Double haploid plant

Answers

1	(a)	25	(a)	49	(d)	73	(a)
2	(a)	26	(d)	50	(c)	74	(a)
3	(a)	27	(d)	51	(d)	75	(d)
4	(a)	28	(a)	52	(c)	76	(b)
5	(a)	29	(c)	53	(a)	77	(c)
6	(a)	30	(b)	54	(b)	78	(d)
7	(d)	31	(a)	55	(b)	79	(b)
8	(d)	32	(d)	56	(c)	80	(a)
9	(a)	33	(b)	57	(a)	81	(a)
10	(d)	34	(c)	58	(c)	82	(a)
11	(b)	35	(a)	59	(b)	83	(b)
12	(c)	36	(d)	60	(c)	84	(b)
13	(d)	37	(a)	61	(d)	85	(a)
14	(a)	38	(c)	62	(a)	86	(a)
15	(c)	39	(c)	63	(c)	87	(a)
16	(a)	40	(c)	64	(d)	88	(d)
17	(a)	41	(a)	65	(c)	89	(a)
18	(c)	42	(d)	66	(d)	90	(b)
19	(c)	43	(c)	67	(b)	91	(b)
20	(a)	44	(d)	68	(a)	92	(a)
21	(c)	45	(c)	69	(c)	93	(d)
22	(d)	46	(b)	70	(b)	94	(b)
23	(a)	47	(b)	71	(a)	95	(d)
24	(b)	48	(a)	72	(c)	96	(d)

97	**(c)**	**111**	**(c)**	**125**	**(c)**	**139**	**(c)**
98	**(d)**	**112**	**(a)**	**126**	**(a)**	**140**	**(d)**
99	**(a)**	**113**	**(c)**	**127**	**(b)**	**141**	**(d)**
100	**(d)**	**114**	**(d)**	**128**	**(b)**	**142**	**(d)**
101	**(a)**	**115**	**(c)**	**129**	**(b)**	**143**	**(a)**
102	**(b)**	**116**	**(d)**	**130**	**(b)**	**144**	**(b)**
103	**(b)**	**117**	**(c)**	**131**	**(a)**	**145**	**(c)**
104	**(c)**	**118**	**(c)**	**132**	**(a)**	**146**	**(b)**
105	**(a)**	**119**	**(c)**	**133**	**(d)**	**147**	**(b)**
106	**(c)**	**120**	**(c)**	**134**	**(b)**	**148**	**(c)**
107	**(a)**	**121**	**(c)**	**135**	**(a)**	**149**	**(c)**
108	**(b)**	**122**	**(a)**	**136**	**(a)**	**150**	**(a)**
109	**(b)**	**123**	**(c)**	**137**	**(b)**		
110	**(d)**	**124**	**(b)**	**138**	**(a)**		

Chapter 29
Plant Cell Culture

1. **Protoplasts are the cells devoid of**
   (a) Cell membrane
   (b) Cell wall
   (c) Both cell wall and cell membrane
   (d) None of these

2. **Protoplasts can be produced from suspension cultures, callus tissues or intact tissues by enzymatic treatment with**
   (a) Cellulotyic enzymes
   (b) Pectolytic enzymes
   (c) Both cellulotyic and pectolytic enzymes
   (d) Proteolytic enzymes

3. **When plated only in nutrient medium, how much time is required for the protoplast to synthesize new cell wall?**
   (a) 2-5 days
   (b) 5-10 days
   (c) 10-15 days
   (d) 15-17 days

4. **In a callus culture**
   (a) Increasing level of cytokinin to a callus induces shoot formation and increasing level of auxin promote root formation
   (b) Increasing level of auxin to a callus induces shoot formation and increasing level of cytokinin promote root formation
   (c) Auxins and cytokinins are not required
   (d) Only auxin is required for root and shoot formation

5. **Organogenesis is**
   (a) Formation of callus tissue
   (b) Formation of root and shoots on callus tissue
   (c) Both (a) and (b)
   (d) Genesis of organs

6. **Which breeding method uses a chemical to strip the cell wall of plant cells of two sexually incompatible species?**
   (a) Mass selection (b) Protoplast fusion
   (c) Transformation (d) Transpiration

7. **Which method of plant propagation involves the use of girdling?**
   (a) Grafting (b) Cuttings
   (c) Layering (d) Micropropagation

8. **A (n) _________ is an excised piece of leaf or stein tissue used in micropropagation.**
   (a) Microshoot (b) Medium
   (c) Extant (d) Scion

9. **Subculturing is similar to propagation by cuttings because**
   (a) It separates multiple microshoots and places them in a medium
   (b) It uses scions to produce new microshoots
   (c) They both use in vitro growing conditions
   (d) All of the above

10. **Cell fusion method includes the preparation of**
   (a) Plant cells stripped of their cell wall
   (b) Single plant cell stripped of their cell wall
   (c) Plant cells with cell wall
   (d) Cells from different species

Answers

1	(c)	4	(a)	7	(c)	10	(b)
2	(c)	5	(b)	8	(c)		
3	(b)	6	(b)	9	(a)		

Chapter 30
Plant Cell Culture Media

1. **What are the macronutrients used in plant cell culture medium?**
   (a) N, P, K, S, Na
   (b) N. P, K, Ca, Cl
   (c) N, P, K, S, Ca
   (d) N, P, Ca, Na, CI

2. **Which is the most common carbon source used in the plant cell culture media?**
   (a) Sucrose
   (b) Glucose
   (c) Fructose
   (d) Maltose

3. **Concentration of sucrose generally used in plant cell culture media is**
   (a) 10-15 g/l
   (b) 20-30 g/l
   (c) 40-50 g/l
   (d) 60-70 g/l

4. **Very high sugar concentration (40-100 g/I) have been used**
   (a) In specialized secondary metabolite production
   (b) To adjust the osmotic potential of the media in short term treatment for regeneration
   (c) Both (a) and (b)
   (d) None of these

5. **Which of the following growth regulator cause plant cells to grow?**
   (a) Auxins
   (b) Cytokinins
   (c) Gibberellins
   (d) Brassinosteroids

6. **Which of the following growth regulator promote cell division?**
   (a) Auxins
   (b) Cytokinins
   (c) Gibberellins
   (d) Brassinosteroids

7. **Which of the following growth regulator is added for short initiation during plant regeneration from callus?**
   (a) Auxins
   (b) Cytokinins
   (c) Gibberellins
   (d) Brassinosteroids

8. **Which of the following growth regulator is used to stimulate embryo or shoot development?**
   (a) Auxins
   (b) Cytokinins
   (c) Gibberellins
   (d) Brassinosteroids

9. **Which is/are the naturally occurring plant auxins?**
   (a) Naphthalenacetic acid (NAA)
   (b) Indole acetic acid (IAA)
   (c) 2,4-dichlorophenoxyacetic acid
   (d) All of the above

10. **Which is/are the disadvantage/(s) of using IAA in plant cell culture media?**
   (a) It is unstable in solution
   (b) Gets easily oxidized
   (c) Conjugated to inactive form by plant cells
   (d) All of the above

11. **Which of the following is not an auxin?**
   (a) Naphthalenacetic acid (NAA)
   (b) Indole acetic acid (IAA)
   (c) Zeatin
   (d) Indole butyric acid

12. **Which of the following is not a cytokinin?**
   (a) 2,4-dichlorophenoxyacetic acid
   (b) 6-benzylaminopurine
   (c) Zeatin
   (d) Kinetin

13. **In plant cell culture media, auxins and cytokinins are used in the range of**
   (a) 1-50μM
   (b) 50-100μM
   (c) 100-125μM
   (d) More than 125μM

14. **Nitrogen in the plant cell culture media is provided by either ammonia or nitrate salt. In the media**
   (a) Utilization of ammonium cause culture pH to drop while utilization of nitrate cause culture pH to rise
   (b) Utilization of nitrate cause culture pH to drop while utilization of ammonium cause culture pH to rise
   (c) Utilization of both ammonium and nitrate result in rise in pH
   (d) Utilization of both ammonium and nitrate result in drop in pH

15. **To maintain the pH of the culture**
   (a) Organic acid such as citric, fumaric, malic and succinic acid is used
   (b) Synthetic buffers such as Tris, MES or HEPS are used
   (c) Both (a) and (b)
   (d) Ammonium salts are used

16. Neutralized activated charcoal is occasionally added to young re-generating cultures to

(a) Remove toxic phenolics produced by the stressed plant cell

(b) Help to remove plants growth regulators introduced at an earlier stage

(c) Both (a) and (b)

(d) Maintain the pH of the medium

17. Which of the following is an ethylene biosynthesis inhibitor?

(a) Citric acid (b) Succinic acid

(c) Activated charcoal (d) Silver thiosulphate

18. Silver thiosulphate is added to culture medium as it helps to

(a) Maintain the pH

(b) Remove toxic phenolics from plant cells

(c) Prevent the gaseous plant hormone, ethylene dioxide from accumulating to detrimental condition

(d) All of the above

19. What is 'nurse' or conditioned medium?

(a) It is the media full of growth factors used for the growth of cells

(b) It is the medium added to nurse the callus culture

(c) Both (a) and (b)

(d) It is the liquid medium removed from the suspension of fast growing cells

20. Which of the following is not true about nurse or conditioned medium?

(a) It is liquid removed from the suspension of fast growing cells

(b) It contains uncharacterized growth factor released by growing cells

(c) It is used in the culture of regenerating protoplast

(d) It is removed aseptically from the culture and is autoclaved before use

Answers

1	(c)	6	(b)	11	(c)	16	(c)
2	(a)	7	(b)	12	(a)	17	(d)
3	(b)	8	(c)	13	(a)	18	(c)
4	(c)	9	(b)	14	(a)	19	(d)
5	(a)	10	(d)	15	(c)	20	(d)

Chapter 31
Gene Transfer in Plants

1. ***Agrobacterium tumefaciens* is a**
   (a) Gram (+) bacteria
   (b) Gram (-) bacteria
   (c) A fungi
   (d) A yeast

2. **Which of the following is true about *Agrobacterium tumefaciens*?**
   (a) It causes crown gall disease of plants
   (b) It infects gymnosperms
   (c) It infects dicotyledonous angiosperms
   (d) All of the above

3. **Crown gall tissue**
   (a) Can be cultivated in vitro in absence of bacteria
   (b) Retains tumorous properties when cultivated
   (c) Both (a) and (b)
   (d) Shows tumorous properties only in presence of bacteria

4. **Opines are**
   (a) Amino acid derivatives found in tumor tissues
   (b) Amino acid derivatives found in normal tissues
   (c) Amino acid derivatives found in both normal as well as tumor tissues
   (d) None of the above

5. **Opines that are present in crown gall tumour include**
   (a) Octopine
   (b) Nopaline
   (c) Agropine
   (d) All of these

6. **Opine synthesis is the property**
   (a) Conferred to plant cells when it transformed by *Agrobacterium tumefaciens*
   (b) Determined by the bacteria *Agrobacterium tumefaciens*
   (c) Both (a) and (b)
   (d) Of normal plant cells

7. **Virulence trait of *Agrobacterium tumefaciens* is borne on**
   (a) Chromosomal DNA
   (b) Tumour inducing plasmid DNA
   (c) Both chromosomal and plasmid DNA
   (d) Cryptic plasmid DNA

8. **The size of the virulent plasmid of *Agrobacterium tumefaciens* is**
   (a) 40-80 kb (b) 80-120kb
   (c) 140-235kb (d) > 235kb

9. **In a plant tumour cell**
   (a) Complete Ti plasmid is incorporated in plant nuclear DNA
   (b) Different parts of the Ti-plasmid are incorporated
   (c) Only a small specific segment of callus T DNA is incorporated
   (d) May vary from plant to plant

10. **Which of the following is true about T DNA?**
   (a) Integration of T DNA can occur at many different, apparently random, sites in the plant nuclear DNA
   (b) Integration of T DNA occurs only at one specific sites in the plant nuclear DNA
   (c) Integration of T DNA occurs at two specific sites in the plant nuclear DNA
   (d) Integration of T DNA occurs at one site that may be random in the plant nuclear DNA

11. **Integrated nopaline T-DNA occurs as**
   (a) Single segment (b) Two segments
   (c) Three segments (d) Four segments

12. **Integrated octopine T DNA occurs as**
   (a) Single segment (b) Two segments
   (c) Three segments (d) Four segments

13. **The left segment of octopine T-DNA (TL) is necessary for**
   (a) Enzymes for agropine biosynthesis (b) Tumour formation
   (c) Conjugative transfer (d) All of these

14. **The right segment of octopine T-DNA (TR) is necessary for**
   (a) Enzymes for agropine biosynthesis (b) Tumour formation
   (c) Conjugative transfer (d) All of these

15. On Ti-plasmid T-region or T-DNA is flanked by a direct repeat of

(a) I2 by (b) 20 bp

(c) 25 bp (d) 30 bp

16. The direct repeats flanking the T-DNA of *Agrobacterium tumefaciens* are known as

(a) Cos site (b) Flanking sequences

(c) Border sequences (d) Transfer sequences

17. Which of the following is not true about the direct repeats flanking T-DNA?

(a) They are conserved between nopaline and octopine Ti-plasmids

(b) These repeats are transferred intact to the plant genome

(c) These are important in integration mechanism

(d) All of the above

18. T-DNA transfer and processing into plant genome requires products of which of the following genes?

(a) *Vir* A,B (b) *Vir* G,C

(c) *Vir* D, E (d) All of these

19. Vir genes required for the T-DNA transfer and processing are located

(a) On the T-DNA (b) Outside the T-DNA region

(c) On the plant genome (d) None of these

20. Which of the following plant signal molecules regulate the expression of vir B, C, D and E in case of tobacco?

(a) Acetosyringone (b) A-hydroxy syringone

(c) Both (a) and (b) (d) None of these

21. Which of the following genes are constitutively expressed and control the plant induced activation of other vir genes?

(a) *Vir* A and *vir* G (b) *Vir* C and *vir* D

(c) *Vir* B and *vir* E (d) *Vir* A and *vir* B

22. In response to the activating signal molecule, an endonuclease is produced that causes nicks in the T-DNA. It is encoded by

(a) *Vir* A (b) *Vir* B

(c) *Vir* C (d) *Vir* D

23. Because of large size of Ti-plasmid, intermediate vectors (IV) are developed in which T DNA has been subcloned into

(a) PBR 322 based plasmid vector (b) PRK 2013

(c) PRN 3 (d) All of these

24. Intermediate vectors containing T-DNA are conjugation deficient. Thus conjugation is mediated in presence of which of the following plasmid?

(a) PRK 2013 (b) PRN 3

(c) Either (a) or (b) (d) None of these

25. Which of the following is not true about the helper plasmids?

(a) These can replicate in Agrobacterium

(b) These help in the mediating conjugation of intermediate vectors

(c) These can't replicate in Agrobacterium

(d) All of the above

26. The transfer of intermediate vectors into Agrobacterium are brought about by

(a) Transformation (b) Biparental mating

(c) Triparental mating (d) Transduction

27. Which of the following are used as selection marker for the cells transformed with Agrobacterium?

(a) Neomycin phosphotransferase

(b) Streptomycin phosphotransferase

(c) Hygromycin phosphotransferase

(d) Any of the above

28. Direct DNA uptake by protoplasts can be stimulated by

(a) Polyethylene glycol (PEG) (b) Decanal

(c) Luciferin (d) All of these

29. Which of the following is not true for microinjection technique that involves transfer of DNA into protoplast?

(a) It is carried out with the help of micromanipulator

(b) The recipient cells are immobilized on artificial support or artificially bound to substarate

(c) It employs needle with diameter greater than cell diameter

(d) All of the above

30. Microinjection involves

(a) Injection of large amount of DNA

(b) Injection of DNA into bigger cells

(c) Injection with needle having diameter greater than cell diameter

(d) All of the above

31. Microprojectile method of gene transfer in plants involves delivery of DNA

(a) With the help of micromanipulator

(b) With the help of bolistics

(c) With the help of needles

(d) Any of the above

32. Advantage of microprojectile method over microinjection method for gene transfer in plants include

(a) Intact cells are used

(b) Method is universal in its application irrespective of all shape, size, type and presence or absence of cell wall

(c) Gene can be transferred to many cells simultaneously

(d) All of the above

33. Liposomes mediated gene transfer in plants involves

(a) Plasmid DNA enclosed in a lipid bag

(b) Fusion of liposomes with protoplast

(c) Use of polyethylene glycol (PEG)

(d) All of the above

34. In the liposome mediated gene transfer in plants, nucleic acids are

(a) Protected from nuclease digestion

(b) Stable in liposomes

(c) Both (a) and (b)

(d) Not stable in liposomes

35. Plant transformation vectors based on Agrobacterium can generally be divided into

(a) Two vectors

(b) Four vectors

(c) Six vectors

(d) Eight vectors

36. Co-integrating transformation vectors must include a region of homology in

(a) The vector plasmid

(b) The Ti-plasmid

(c) Between vector plasmid and Ti-plasmid

(d) None of these

37. Virulent strains of Agrobacterium contain large Ti-plasmids, which are responsible for the DNA transfer and subsequent disease symptoms. It has been shown that Ti-plasmids contain

(a) One set of sequence necessary for gene transfer

(b) Two sets of sequence necessary for gene transfer

(c) Three sets of sequence necessary for gene transfer

(d) Four sets of sequence necessary for gene transfer

38. Which technique is used to introduce genes into dicots?

(a) Electroporation (b) Particle acceleration

(c) Microinjection (d) Ti plasmid infection

Answers

1	(b)	11	(a)	21	(a)	31	(b)
2	(d)	12	(b)	22	(d)	32	(d)
3	(c)	13	(b)	23	(a)	33	(d)
4	(a)	14	(a)	24	(c)	34	(c)
5	(d)	15	(c)	25	(a)	35	(a)
6	(c)	16	(c)	26	(c)	36	(c)
7	(b)	17	(b)	27	(d)	37	(b)
8	(c)	18	(d)	28	(a)	38	(d)
9	(c)	19	(b)	29	(c)		
10	(a)	20	(c)	30	(c)		

Chapter 32
Transgenic Plants

1. **The first transgenic plants expressing engineered foreign genes were tobacco plants produced by the use of**
   (a) *Agrobacterium tumefaciens*
   (b) *Bacillus thuringiensis*
   (c) *Arabidopsis thaliana*
   (d) *Streptomyces hygroscopicus*

2. **For developing herbicide resistance in transgenic plants which of the following approach/(es) is/are used?**
   (a) Target molecule is made insensitive to herbicide
   (b) Target protein is overproduced
   (c) A pathway should be introduced that detoxify the herbicide
   (d) All of the above

3. **Resistance to glyphosphate in transgenic petunia plants has been developed by the transfer of**
   (a) Gene for EPSPS(5-enol-pyruvyl shikimat 3 phosphate synthase)
   (b) Gene for ALS (acetolactate synthase)
   (c) Gene for GS (glutamine synthase)
   (d) Any of the above

4. **Resistance to sulphonyl urea compounds in transgenic tobacco plant has been developed by the transfer of**
   (a) Gene for EPSPS (5-enol-pyruvyl shikimat 3 phosphate synthase)
   (b) Gene for ALS (acetolactate synthase)
   (c) Gene for GS (glutamine synthase)
   (d) Any of the above

5. **Resistance to L-phosphinothrium in tobacco plants is developed by the transfer of**
   (a) Gene for EPSPS (5-enol-pyruvyl shikimat 3 phosphate synthase)
   (b) Gene for ALS (acetolactate synthase)
   (c) Gene for GS (glutamine synthase)
   (d) Any of the above

6. **Which of the following gene is transferred to plants that detoxify the herbicide atrazine?**
   (a) Nitrilase
   (b) Glutathione S-transferase (GST)
   (c) Phosphinothrium acetyl transferase
   (d) All of these

7. **Which of the following gene detoxify herbicide bronoxynil?**
   (a) Nitrilase
   (b) Glutathione S-transferase (GST)
   (c) Phosphinothricin acetyl transferase
   (d) All of these

8. **Which of the following gene detoxifies herbicide phosphinothricin?**
   (a) Nitrilase
   (b) Glutathione S-transferase (GST)
   (c) Phosphinothricin acetyl transferase
   (d) All of these

9. **Fusion of karyoplast with the enucleated cell is achieved in presence of**
   (a) Cytochalasin B
   (b) Polyethylene glycol
   (c) Both (a) and (b)
   (d) Alcohol

10. **Transfection refers to which of the following?**
    (a) Synthesis of mRNA from DNA template
    (b) Synthesis of protein based on mRNA sequence
    (c) Introduction of foreign gene in to a cell
    (d) The process by which a cell become malignant

11. **Which of the following is/are the method of transfection for making transgenic animals?**
    (a) Transfer or whole nuclei
    (b) Transfer of whole individual chromosomes or fragment
    (c) Transfer of DNA
    (d) All of the above

12. For the transfer of whole individual chromosomes, they are isolated from the cells at

(a) Prophase
(b) Metaphase
(c) Telophase
(d) Anaphase

13. Chromosomes may be isolated from metaphase cells by

(a) Hyportonic lysis
(b) Hypotonic lysis
(c) Either (a) or (b)
(d) Isotonic lysis

14. DNA is microinfected into the fertilized egg

(a) After the fusion of male and female nuclei
(b) Before the fusion of male and female nuclei
(c) At the time of fusion of male and female nuclei
(d) Any time, it can be infected

15. DNA microinjection into the egg has been used to produce which of the following transgenic animals?

(a) Mice
(b) Chicken
(c) Pigs
(d) All of these

16. Animal pharming can be defined as

(a) Growing animals for farming
(b) Programming animals to produce novel products
(c) Generating transgenic animals for farming
(d) None of the above

17. Which protein has been produced generating a transgenic sheep that is used for replacement therapy for individuals at risk from emphysema?

(a) Plasminogen activator (tPA)
(b) α-anti trypsin (AAT)
(c) Casein
(d) Amyloid precursor proteins

18. Transgenic goats have been used to produce which of the following protein that is used for dissolving blood clots?

(a) Amyloid precursor protein
(b) α_1-anti trypsin (AAT)
(d) The process by which a cell become malignant
(c) Casein

19. Transgenic goats produce a variant of human tissue type plasminogen activator protein in

(a) Blood
(b) Urine
(c) Milk
(d) Muscles

20. In transgenic fish, the genes are introduced by

(a) Microinjection in fish
(b) Viruses
(c) Transfer of whole nuclei
(d) All of these

21. Which of the following gene have been introduced into the transgenic fish?

(a) Human or rat gene for growth hormone
(b) Chicken gene for delta crystalline protein
(c) *E. coli* gene for β-galactosidase
(d) All of the above

22. DNA into fish is injected into

(a) Pronuclei
(b) Cytoplasm
(c) Both (a) and (b)
(d) None of these

Answers

1	(a)	7	(a)	13	(b)	19	(c)
2	(d)	8	(c)	14	(b)	20	(a)
3	(a)	9	(b)	15	(d)	21	(d)
4	(b)	10	(c)	16	(b)	22	(b)
5	(c)	11	(d)	17	(b)		
6	(b)	12	(b)	18	(d)		

Chapter 33
Immune Chemistry

Monoclonal Antibodies

1. **In monoclonal antibody technology, tumor cells that can replicate endlessly are fused with mammalian cells that produce an antibody. The result of this cell fusion is a**
   (a) Hybridoma
   (b) Myeloma
   (c) Natural killer cell
   (d) Lymphoblast

2. **T cells are the source of**
   (a) Interleukin
   (b) Interferon
   (c) Lymphotoxin
   (d) All of these

3. **Some cross reactions with monoclonal antibodies (MAbs) can occur. Unexpected cross reactions occur more frequently with**
   (a) Ig MAbs
   (b) IgG
   (c) IgA
   (d) IgE

4. **The primary B cell receptor is**
   (a) IgD
   (b) IgG
   (c) IgA
   (d) 1gE

5. **The antigen-specific lymphocytes can be immortalized by which of the following method?**
   (a) Transfection with tumor derived DNA
   (b) Hybridization with a suitable lymphoid tumor cell
   (c) Transformation following infection by Epstein-Barr virus (EBV)
   (d) All of the above

6. **Small simple molecules are**
   (a) Poor antigens
   (b) Rich antigens
   (c) Moderate antigens
   (d) Heterophilic antigens

7. **It is highly valued if the lymphocytes derived from the lymph node or tonsil tend to undergo fusion at**
   (a) High frequencies
   (b) Moderate frequencies
   (c) Low frequencies
   (d) At no frequency

8. **Which type of cell actually secrets antibodies?**
   (a) Plasma cells
   (b) T cells
   (c) Macrophages
   (d) Dendritic cells

9. **The approach (s), which is/are currently followed to produce human monoclonal antibodies, is/are known as**
   (a) Transformation of antigen specific B lymphocytes (EBV)
   (b) Hybridization of 6-thioguanine-resistant human plasmacytoma with immune human lymphocytes
   (c) Combination of EBVand hybridoma techniques
   (d) All of these

10. **An example of mosaic antigen is**
   (a) Virus
   (b) Bacteria
   (c) A hapten
   (d) Protein

11. **In human B cells and T cells are matured in the**
   (a) Bone marrow and thymus respectively
   (b) Lymph nodes and spleen respectively
   (c) Bursa and thymus respectively
   (d) None of these

12. **The EBV-hybridoma technique**
   (a) Immortalizes the donor Bcells
   (b) Facilitates the proliferation of antigen specific B cells
   (c) Gives much higher hybridization frequencies
   (d) All of the above

13. **The cross linkage of antigens by antibodies is known as**
   (a) Agglutination
   (b) Complement fixation
   (c) A cross reaction
   (d) All of these

14. **A cytokine that stimulates the activity of B and T cells is**
   (a) Lymphotoxin
   (b) Interlukin-2
   (c) Interlukin-1
   (d) All of these

15. In immuno-inflammatory diseases such as haemolytic anaemia, eczema etc.,

(a) T8 cells are greatly reduced
(b) T8 cells are greatly increased
(c) T4 cells are greatly reduced
(d) T4 cells are greatly increased

16. Helper T cells assist in the functions of

(a) Certain B cells
(b) Certain T cells
(c) Certain B cells and other T cells
(d) None of the above

17. The hybrid cells can be propagated

(a) In tissue culture
(b) As ascites in peritoneal cavity of mice
(c) Both (a) and (b)
(d) None of these

18. T_C cells are important in controlling

(a) Virus infections
(b) Allergy
(c) Autoimmunity
(d) All of these

19. Preliminary clinical results with a humanized antibody against the interleukin-2 receptor have suggested the

(a) Absence of human immune response against murine proteins (HAMA) response
(b) Presence of HAMA response
(c) Poor recognition of immunoglobulin, Ig constant regions
(d) All of the above

Answers

1	(a)	6	(a)	11	(a)	16	(c)
2	(c)	7	(a)	12	(d)	17	(c)
3	(a)	8	(a)	13	(a)	18	(d)
4	(a)	9	(d)	14	(b)	19	(a)
5	(d)	10	(a)	15	(a)		

Chapter 34
Immunology

1. **Antibodies are**
   (a) Proteins
   (b) Glycoproteins
   (c) Carbohydrates
   (d) Nucleic acid

2. **Antibodies consists of**
   (a) 2 light chains and 2 heavy chains arranged in a Y-shaped configuration
   (b) A light chain and 2 heavy chains arranged in a Y-shaped configuration
   (c) 2 light chains and a heavy chain arranged in a Y-shaped configuration
   (d) All of these

3. **Light chains and heavy chains are joined together by**
   (a) Covalent bond
   (b) Hydrogen bond
   (c) Di-sulphide bond
   (d) Ionic bond

4. **Antigen binding site on an antibody is known as**
   (a) Antitope
   (b) Epitope
   (c) Paratope
   (d) Endotope

5. **An antibody has**
   (a) 2 Fab regions and an Fc region
   (b) An Fab region and an Fc region
   (c) 2 Fab regions and 2 Fc regions
   (d) many Fab regions and many Fc regions

6. **Hypervariable region resides in the**
   (a) N terminal region of light chain
   (b) N-terminal region of light and heavy chain
   (c) C-terminal region of light chain
   (d) C-terminal region of light chain and heavy chain

7. **Fab stands for the following**
   (a) Fragment antibody binding
   (b) Fragment antigen binding
   (c) Fragment antibody or antigen binding
   (d) Fragment affinity binding

8. **Which of the following statement is true for the Fc region**
   (a) Fragment crystalisation and is the constant region
   (b) Fragment constant and is the variable region
   (c) Fragment crystalisation and is the variable region
   (d) Fragment crystalisation and has both variable and constant region

9. **Fab region has a**
   (a) Hypervariable region that binds with antibody
   (b) Hypervariable region that binds with antigen
   (c) Hypervariable region that binds with other immune cells
   (d) All of th above

10. **Fc region is involved in**
   (a)
   Cell surface receptor binding
   (b) Complement activation
   (c) Determining diffusivity of antibody molecule
   (d) All of the above

11. **Ability of antigen to stimulate antibody production is called**
   (a) Affinity
   (b) Antigenicity
   (c) Elicitation
   (d) None of these

12. **Light chains and heavy chains of antibodies are joined by**
   (a) Hydrogen bond
   (b) Hydrophobic bond
   (c) Di-sulphide bond
   (d) Ionic bond

13. **Clearance of antigens by antibodies involve**
   (a) Neutralization and agglutination
   (b) Opsonisation and complement activation
   (c) Precipitation
   (d) All of the above

14. **Two identical light chains of an antibody belongs to**
   (a) Kappa only
   (b) Lambda only
   (c) Lambda or kappa
   (d) None of the above

15. Hypervariable region of antibody consists of

(a) 5-10 aminoacids that form antigen binding site
(b) 50-100 aminoacids that form antigen binding site
(c) 5-10 aminoacids that forms the antibody binding site
(d) A part of constant region of heavy and light chain

16. Which of the following is the most abundant immunoglobulin (Ig)

(a) IgM (b) IgG
(c) IgA (d) IgE

17. Which of the following IgG is targeted against polysaccharides of encapsulated bacteria

(a) IgG1 (b) IgG2
(c) IgG3 (d) IgG4

18. IgG consists of

(a) 2 light chains and two heavy chains joined by di-sulphide bond (H2L2)
(b) 2 light chains and two heavy chains joined by hydrogen bond (H2L2)
(c) 2 light chains and a heavy chain joined by di-sulphide bond (H1L2)
(d) A light chain and two heavy chains joined by di-sulphide bond (H2L1)

19. Which is the Ig that can cross placenta and provide passive immunity to new born

(a) IgM (b) IgG
(c) IgA (d) IgE

20. Which is the Ig that first reaches the site of infection

(a) IgM (b) IgG
(c) IgA (d) IgE

21. Which is the largest Ig

(a) IgM (b) IgG
(c) IgA (d) IgE

22. Which of the following statements are true regarding IgM

(a) IgM is a pentamer and is the largest Ig and called as 'natural antibody'
(b) IgM exists as monomer on B-cell surface
(c) IgM is involved in early primary immune response
(d) All of the above

23. Which of the following statements are true

(a) IgM is involved in primary immune response

(b) IgG is involved in primary immune response

(c) Both IgM and IgG are involved in primary immune response

(d) IgG is involved only in secondary immune response

24. Antibody present in secretions like tears, saliva, colostrum is

(a) IgM (b) IgG

(c) IgA (d) IgE

25. Primary Ig of exocrine secretions is

(a) IgM (b) IgG

(c) IgA (d) IgE

26. Second most abundant Ig is

(a) IgM (b) IgG

(c) IgA (d) IgE

27. Most effective Ig is

(a) IgM (b) IgG

(c) IgA (d) IgE

28. IgM is a

(a) Pentamer with 10 antigen binding sites

(b) Tetramer with 8 antigen binding sites

(c) Monomer with 2 antigen binding sites

(d) Dimer with 4 antigen binding sites

29. Ig that mediates allergic reaction is

(a) IgM (b) IgG

(c) IgA (d) IgE

30. Ig involved in host defence against parasitic infection (helminths)

(a) IgM (b) IgG

(c) IgA (d) IgE

31. Any substance or molecules that interact with antibodies are called

(a) Antigens (b) Antibodies

(c) Epitope (d) Immunogens

32. Antigens can be

(a) Proteins (b) Carbohydrates

(c) Nucleic acids (d) All of these

51. Stomach clear out pathogens by

(a) Secreting HCl
(b) Secreting digestive enzymes
(c) Both (a) and (b)
(d) None of these

52. Vaginal bacterial symbionts like Lactobacilli prevents pathogen by

(a) Producing lactic acid thereby reducing pH
(b) Secreting antibiotics
(c) Secreting toxins
(d) None of these

53. Bodies internal defence or second line of defence include

(a) Phagocytes
(b) Fever
(c) Interferons
(d) All of the above

54. Functions of macrophages include

(a) Phagocytosis
(b) Antigen presenting cells
(c) Cytokine production
(d) All of the above

55. Kupffer cells are macrophages found on

(a) Lung
(b) Bone
(c) Nephrons
(d) Liver

56. Neutrophils are

(a) Phagocytes
(b) Short lived leucocytes
(c) Involved in second line of defence
(d) All of the above

57. Tissue damage caused by wound or invading pathogenic organisms induces a complex sequence of events collectively known as

(a) Opsonisation
(b) Phagocytosis
(c) Inflammation
(d) None of the above

58. Temperature rising chemicals are called

(a) Pyrogens
(b) Thermogens
(c) Both a and b
(d) None of these

59. Internal second line of defence involves all except

(a) Natural killer cells
(b) Complement system
(c) Interferons
(d) Antibodies

60. Antiviral glycoproteins released by living cells in response to viral attack and induce a viral resistant state to neighbouring cells is called as

(a) Natural killer cells
(b) Complement system
(c) Interferons
(d) Phagocytes

61. Humoral immunity is mediated by

(a) B cells
(b) Macrophages
(c) Both (a) and (b)
(d) Phagocytes

62. Humoral immunity is also called as

(a) Antibody mediated immunity
(b) Non-specific immune response
(c) Antigen mediated immunity
(d) All of these

63. B cell has receptor on its surface which is

(a) Monomeric IgM
(b) Dimeric IgM
(c) Monomeric IgG
(d) B cell receptor

64. B cells upon activation by antigens

(a) Undergo clonal expansion followed by clonal selection
(b) Divides continuously
(c) Undergo clonal selection followed by clonal expansion
(d) Secrete antibodies

65. B cells differentiates to form

(a) Plasma cells
(b) Effector cells
(c) Plasma cells and memory B cells
(d) None of these

66. Which of the following statement is incorrect regarding plasma cells

(a) Plasma cells are the effector cells
(b) Plasma cells secretes antibodies
(c) The precursor of plasma cell is B cell
(d) Plasma cell has surface receptors

67. Origin and maturation of B cells takes place at

(a) Spleen
(b) Thymus
(c) Bone marrow
(d) Lymph nodes

68. The function of memory B cell is

(a) Antibody production
(b) Immunologic memory
(c) Regulated antibody production
(d) None of these

69. B cells are

(a) Lymphocytes which are short lived
(b) Lymphocytes which are long lived

(c) Lymphocytes involved in non-specific defence
(d) None of these

70. Generally antibodies produced against a pathogen is
(a) Monoclonal
(b) Homogenous
(c) Polyclonal
(d) All of same specificity

71. Antibodies produced by plasma cells are
(a) Specific
(b) Produced against the epitope that triggered B cell activation
(c) Both (a) and (b)
(d) Diverse

72. Antibodies clear out antigens by
(a) Neutralization
(b) Precipitation
(c) Agglutination
(d) All of these

73. Antibodies are
(a) Opsonins
(b) Lipoproteins
(c) Serum phagocytes
(d) None of these

74. Any substance that promotes phagocytosis of antigens by binding to them are called as
(a) Opsonins
(b) Phagocytes
(c) Macrophages
(d) Interleukins

75. The phenomenon of selective proliferation of B cells in response to their interaction with the antigen is called
(a) Clonal expansion
(b) Monoclonal selection
(c) Clonal proliferation
(d) Clonal selection

76. The specific targeted responses constitute the third line of defence in response to an infectious agent and is called as
(a) Third line of defence
(b) Adaptive immunity
(c) Acquired immunity
(d) All of these

77. The characteristics of adaptive immunity include
(a) Specificity
(b) Immunologic memory
(c) Discrimination of self from non self molecules
(d) All of these

78. Which of the cells are involved in adaptive immunity

(a) B cells and T cells
(b) B cells only
(c) T cells only
(d) Macrophages and NK cells

79. T cell mediates

(a) Humoral immunity
(b) Non-specific defence
(c) Cell mediated immunity
(d) None of these

80. The ratio of T cells to B cells is

(a) 3:1
(b) 1:3
(c) 1:1
(d) 1:2

81. The antibody mediated humoral immunity is mediated by

(a) B cells and T cells
(b) B cells
(c) T cells
(d) Macrophages and NK cells

82. T cells and B cells are originated in

(a) Spleen
(b) Thymus
(c) Bone marrow
(d) Lymph nodes

83. Injection of anti-venom against snake bite is an example of

(a) Active immunity
(b) Passive immunity
(c) Non-specific immunity
(d) Phagocytic immunity

84. Which of the following statements are true regarding adaptive immunity

(a) Prior exposure to antigen is essential
(b) Prior exposure to antigen is not essential
(c) It is a non-specific defence mechanism
(d) Macrophages are the major cells involved

85. Active immunity involves

(a) Contact with foreign antigens
(b) Immunologic memory
(c) Slow primary response
(d) All of the above

86. Active immunity is produced by

(a) Clonal selection
(b) Clonal expansion
(c) Both (a) and (b)
(d) All of these

87. Cells involved in adaptive immunity or acquired immunity or specific defence include

(a) T cells
(b) B cells
(c) Antigen presenting cells
(d) All of these

88. **Plasma cells are secreted by**
(a) T cells (b) B cells
(c) Antigen presenting cells (d) Macrophages

89. **The characteristics of passive immunity include**
(a) Immediate relief (b) No immunologic memory
(c) Resistance for a short period only (d) All of these

90. **Immunologic memory is provided by**
(a) B cells (b) T cells
(c) Both a and b (d) Phagocytes

91. **Immune disorders include**
(a) Hypersensitivity (b) Auto-immune diseases
(c) Immunodeficiency (d) All of these

92. **The inappropriate response of immune system towards a relatively harmless antigen causing harm to the host is referred as**
(a) Hypersensitivity (b) Auto-immune diseases
(c) Immunodeficiency (d) Tolerance

93. **Which of the following Ig is involved in mediating allergic reactions**
(a) IgG (b) IgM
(c) IgE (d) IgA

94. **The major chemical messenger involved in hypersensitivity is**
(a) Interleukines (b) Lymphokines
(c) Hiatamines (d) Interferons

95. **Which of the following types of hypersensitive reactions is antibody mediated**
(a) Type I (b) Type II
(c) Type III (d) All of these

96. **Which one of the following is a cell mediated hypersensitive reaction**
(a) Type I (b) Type II
(c) Type III (d) Type IV

97. **The inability to distinguish between self-cells and non-self-cells may lead to**
(a) Hypersensitivity (b) Auto-immune diseases
(c) Immunodeficiency (d) Tolerance

98. **Majority of auto immune diseases are**
(a) Cell mediated (b) Antibody mediated
(c) Macrophage mediated (d) Mast cells mediated

99. All of the following are autoimmune disorders except

(a) Graves disease
(b) SCID
(c) Rheumatoid arthritis
(d) Addison's disease

100. Rheumatoid arthritis mostly occur in individuals carrying

(a) HLA-DR4 gene (HLA-human leucocyte antigen)
(b) HLA-DR1 gene
(c) HLA-DR3 gene
(d) All of the above

101. Some defects or mutations in components of innate or adaptive immunity may lead to

(a) Hypersensitivity
(b) Auto-immune diseases
(c) Immunodeficiency
(d) Tolerance

102. In severe combined immune deficiency (SCID), the patients are deficient in

(a) B cells
(b) T cells
(c) Both (a) and (b)
(d) IgA

103. SCID can occur due to the absence of an enzyme

(a) Adenosine deaminase
(b) Guanosine deaminase
(c) Phosphorylase
(d) Thymidine deaminase

104. HIV attacks

(a) T helper cells
(b) T cytotoxic cells
(c) B cells
(d) Macrophages

105. All of the following are immunodeficiency diseases except

(a) Graves disease
(b) SCID
(c) DiGeorge's syndrome
(d) Hyper IgM syndrome

106. The process of removal and replacement of damaged tissues or organs with healthy ones from a donor is called as

(a) Transplantation
(b) Replacement therapy
(c) Repair and replacement
(d) None of these

107. The transfer of individuals own tissue to another part of the body is called

(a) Autograft
(b) Xenograft
(c) Allograft
(d) Syngeneic graft

108. The transfer of tissue between genetically identical individuals (like twins) is called

(a) Autograft
(b) Xenograft
(c) Allograft
(d) Syngeneic graft

109. The transfer of tissue between individuals of different species is called

(a) Autograft
(b) Xenograft
(c) Allograft
(d) Syngeneic graft

110. The transfer of tissue between genetically different individuals of same species is called

(a) Autograft
(b) Xenograft
(c) Allograft
(d) Syngeneic graft

111. Which of the following has the maximum transplantation success rate

(a) Autograft
(b) Xenograft
(c) Allograft
(d) Syngeneic graft

112. The major molecules responsible for rejection of transplant is

(a) B cells
(b) T cells
(c) MHC molecule (Major histocompatibility complex)
(d) Antibodies

113. Genes encoding cell surface glycoproteins that are required for antigen presentation to T cells and also responsible for rapid graft rejection is called as

(a) MHC complex
(b) B cell complex
(c) T cell complex
(d) None of these

114. Which of the following statements are true regarding transplantation

(a) The compatibility of MHC proteins of donor and recipient will determine the success of transplantation
(b) MHCs are just like fingerprints and all nucleated cells possess this fingerprint
(c) The compatibility of MHC/HLA proteins of donor and recipient will be high if they are genetically closely related and may lead to successful transplantation.
(d) All of these

115. In humans, MHC is called as

(a) Human MHC
(b) Homo MHC
(c) Human leucocyte antigen (HLA)
(d) All of the above

116. The genes for HLA proteins are clustered in the major histocompatibility complex located

(a) On the short arm of chromosome 6
(b) On the long arm of chromosome 6
(c) On the short arm of chromosome10
(d) On the long arm of chromosome 10

117. The test that is done prior to transplantation surgery to determine the compatibility of MHC proteins between donar and recipient is called

(a) MHC matching (b) MHC typing
(c) Tissue typing (d) Blood HLA test

118. Cyclosporine is an immunosuppressive drug given to avoid transplant rejection which acts by

(a) Inhibition of T cells
(b) Inhibition of B cells
(c) Inhibition of immune system
(d) Inhibition of complement system

119. MHC class I is a cell surface molecule present on

(a) B cells (b) All nucleated cells
(c) APCs (d) T cells

120. MHC class II is a cell surface molecule present on

(a) B cells (b) All nucleated cells
(c) APCs (d) T cells

121. The process of introduction of weakened pathogen into human body is called

(a) Immunization (b) Vaccination
(c) Attenuation (d) None of these

122. The first vaccine was developed by

(a) Louis Pasteur (b) Edward Jenner
(c) Carl Landsteiner (d) Joseph Miester

123. The concept of vaccination was first developed by

(a) Louis Pasteur (b) Edward Jenner
(c) Carl Landsteiner (d) Joseph Miester

124. The process of weakening a pathogen is called

(a) Vaccination (b) Attenuation
(c) Immunization (d) Virulence reduction

125. The first vaccine developed by Louis Pasteur was against

(a) Pox virus (b) Hepatitis virus
(c) Rabies virus (d) None of these

126. A vaccine can be

(a) An antigenic protein (b) Weakened pathogen
(c) Live attenuated pathogen (d) All of these

127. Passive immunisation include

(a) Introduction of antibodies directly

(b) Transfer of maternal antibodies across placenta

(c) Transfer of lymphocyte directly

(d) All of these

128. Which of the following statement is true regarding vaccination

(a) Vaccination is a method of active immunisation

(b) Vaccination is a method of passive immunisation

(c) Vaccination is a method of artificial passive immunisation

(d) Vaccination is a method of natural passive immunization

129. Active immunity may be gained by

(a) Natural infection

(b) Vaccines

(c) Toxoids

(d) All of these

130. Which of the following is a combined vaccine

(a) Hepatitis B vaccine

(b) Hib vaccine

(c) Var vaccine

(d) DPT vaccine

131. The first recombinant antigen vaccine approved for human use is

(a) Hepatitis B vaccine

(b) Hib vaccine

(c) Var vaccine

(d) DPT vaccine

132. Plasmids encoding antigenic protein from a pathogen that is directly injected into the cells where it express constitute

(a) Protein vaccines

(b) Nucleotide vaccines

(c) DNA vaccines

(d) Recombined vaccines

133. All the given vaccines are attenuated or inactivated whole pathogen except

(a) Salk

(b) Sabin

(c) Hepatitis A

(d) Tetanus

134. Which of the following statements are true regarding polio vaccines

(a) Salk and Sabin are polio vaccines

(b) Sabin is live attenuated polio vaccine

(c) Salk is an inactivated polio vaccine

(d) All of these

135. Which of the following is a polysaccharide vaccine

(a) Anthrax vaccine

(b) Rabies vaccine

(c) Hepatitis A

(d) Hib vaccine

136. Complement system
(a) Consists of 20 serum proteins
(b) Serum proteins acts as biological cascade
(c) Both (a) and (b)
(d) Are set of antibodies

137. Complement system is involved in
(a) Specific defence (b) Non-specific defence
(c) Both (a) and (b) (d) None of these

138. Which of the following statements are true regarding complement activation
(a) Lysis of pathogen, tumor cells and allografts
(b) Production of mediators that attracts neutrophils to the site of inflammation
(c) Opsonization
(d) All of these

139. Classical pathway of complement system is activated by
(a) Antibody-antigen complexes (b) Antigen
(c) Antigenic peptides (d) Antigens bound to MHC

140. Alternate pathway of complement system is activated by
(a) Antibody-antigen complexes (b) Antigen
(c) Microorganisms or its toxins (d) Antigens bound to MHC

141. Classical pathway of complement system is involved in
(a) Specific defence (b) Adaptive immunity
(c) Both (a) and (b) (d) Non-specific defence

142. Alternate pathway of complement system is involved in
(a) Non-specific defence (b) Innate immunity
(c) Both (a) and (b) (d) Adaptive immunity

143. Which of the following is the central molecule in complement pathway
(a) C1 (b) C2
(c) C3b (d) C5

144. Cell lysis in complement pathway is initiated by
(a) Membrane destruction complex
(b) Membrane degradation complex
(c) Membrane attacking complex
(d) Membrane lysis complex

145. MAC is

(a) C5b6789 complex
(b) C5b5678 complex
(c) C5b5789 complex
(d) Protein polysaccharide complex

146. Which of the following is required for C1 activation

(a) Ca (b) Mg
(c) Mn (d) Zn

147. Which of the following is the most potent anaphylatoxin

(a) C3a (b) C4a
(c) C5a (d) C1

148. In alternate pathway

(a) Factor b is involved (b) Factor d is involved
(c) Both (a) and (b) (d) Only factor f is involved

149. Biological role of complement system include

(a) Cytolysis and chemotaxis
(b) Opsonisation
(c) Anaphylotoxin and enhanced antibody production
(d) All of these

150. Body's own cells are protected from membrane attack complex by a surface glycoprotein called

(a) MHC (b) DAF
(c) TCR (d) BCR

151. Monoclonal antibodies are

(a) Heterogenous antibodies produced from single clone of plasma cells
(b) Homogenous antibodies produced from single clone of plasma cells
(c) Both (a) and (b)
(d) None of these

152. Natural humoral immune response against a pathogen leads to the production of

(a) Polyclonal antibodies (b) Monoclonal antibodies
(c) Macrophages (d) None of these

153. The technology used for the production of monoclonal antibodies is

(a) Massculture technology (b) Hybridoma technology
(c) Suspension culture (d) None of these

154. Hybridoma technology was developed by

(a) Kohler and Milstein
(b) Khorana and Nirenberg
(c) Khorana and Korenberg
(d) Beedle and Tautum

155. The hybridomas are made by

(a) Fusing T cells with myeloma cells
(b) Fusing B cells with myeloma cells
(c) Fusing T helper cells with myeloma cells
(d) Fusing B memory cells with myeloma cells

156. All are Mabs except

(a) Rituximab
(b) Transtuzumab
(c) Infliximab
(d) Tamoxifen

157. Mabs are

(a) Specific towards a paratope
(b) Specific towards an epitope
(c) Specific towards an antigen
(d) None of these

158. Which of the following statement is incorrect regarding HAT medium

(a) HAT medium is a selective medium
(b) Aminiopterin in the HAT medium blocks de novo pathway of nucleotide synthesis
(c) Salvage pathway requires aminopterin and thymidine
(d) Hypoxanthin is converted to guanine by HGPRT enzyme

159. HGPRT– mutant cells are raised by inducing mutations using

(a) 5-bromouracil
(b) 8-azaguanine
(c) Colchicine
(d) 6-methy isocyanate

160. In hybridoma technology, hybrid cells are selected in

(a) MS medium
(b) HAT medium
(c) X-gal medium
(d) Whites medium

161. Which of the following cell is made deficient of hypoxanthine guanyl phosphoribosyl transferase (HGPRT) enzyme

(a) B cells
(b) Hybrid cells
(c) Myeloma cells
(d) None of these

162. Which of the following statement is incorrect regarding HAT selection

(a) B cells are HGPRT + and can grow in HAT medium but undergoes normal cell death
(b) Myeloma cells cannot grow in HAT medium as these cells lack HGPRT

(c) Hybrid cell survive in HAT medium as it inherits HGPRT form B cells

(d) Aminopterin in HAT medium blocks de novo pathway of nucleotide synthesis only in myeloma cells

163. Mabs are used in

(a) The screening of recombinants
(b) Diagnostic kits
(c) The treatment of many cancers
(d) All of these

164. The major hazards of Mabs are

(a) Difficult in purification
(b) Contamination with retroviral particles from mouse myeloma cells
(c) Non specificity
(d) All of these

165. Mabs are produced by

(a) *In vivo* method
(b) Suspended cell culture in fermenters
(c) Immobilized cell reactors
(d) All of these

166. An antigen is

(a) A highly specific protein produced by the body in response to a foreign body
(b) A chemical that inhibits the growth of micro organisms
(c) An antibody produced by the body that stimulates the production of antibodies by the body's immune system
(d) A chemical substance that stimulates the production of antibodies by the body's immune system

167. CD40 ligand is seen only on

(a) Macrophages
(b) Cytotoxic T cells
(c) Helper T cells
(d) Dentritic cells

168. High titres of antinuclear antibodies are indicative of

(a) Parasitic infections
(b) Fungal diseases
(c) Autoimmune diseases
(d) Bacterial diseases

169. Which of the following is an auto immune disease?

(a) Type 1 Diabetes mellitus
(b) Type 2 Diabetes mellitus
(c) Haemophilia A
(d) Sickle cell anemia

170. DNA vaccines elicit protective immunity against a microbial pathogen by activating:

(a) Humoral immune system
(b) Cellular immune system
(c) Both a) and b)
(d) None of these

171. Which is the first immunoglobulin class to be produced in a primary response to an antigen and also the first immunoglobulin to be synthesised by the neonates:

(a) IgA
(b) IgB
(c) IgD
(d) IgM

172. In an immune response the type of cell which gets activated earliest is:

(a) Killer T cells
(b) Plasma cells
(c) Helper T cells
(d) Cytotoxic T cells

173. What is a characteristic of early stages of local inflammation?

(a) Fever
(b) Anaphylactic Shock
(c) Release of histamine
(d) Attack by cytotoxic T cells

174. An epitope associates with which part of an antibody?

(a) The antibody binding site
(b) The heavy chain constant regions only
(c) Variable regions of a heavy chain and light chain combined
(d) The light chain constant regions only

175. Which of the following is not true about helper T cells?

(a) They function in cell mediated and humoral responses
(b) They are activated by polysaccharide fragments
(c) They bear surface CD4 molecules
(d) They are subject to infection by HIV

176. The specific targeted responses constitute the third line of defence in response to an infectious agent and is called as

(a) Third line of defence
(b) Adaptive immunity
(c) Acquired immunity
(d) All of these

177. The characteristics of adaptive immunity include

(a) Specificity
(b) Immunologic memory
(c) Discrimination of self from non self molecules
(d) All of these

178. Which of the cells are involved in adaptive immunity

(a) B cells and T cells
(b) B cells only
(c) T cells only
(d) Macrophages and NK cells

179. T cell mediates

(a) Humoral immunity
(b) Non-specific defence
(c) Cell mediated immunity
(d) None of these

180. The ratio of T cells to B cells is

(a) 3:1
(b) 1:3
(c) 1:1
(d) 1:2

181. The antibody mediated humoral immunity is mediated by

(a) B cells and T cells
(b) B cells
(c) T cells
(d) Macrophages and NK cells

182. T cells and B cells are originated in

(a) Spleen
(b) Thymus
(c) Bone marrow
(d) Lymph nodes

183. Injection of anti-venom against snake bite is an example of

(a) Active immunity
(b) Passive immunity
(c) Non-specific immunity
(d) Phagocytic immunity

184. Which of the following statements are true regarding adaptive immunity

(a) Prior exposure to antigen is essential
(b) Prior exposure to antigen is not essential
(c) It is a non-specific defence mechanism
(d) Macrophages are the major cells involved

185. Active immunity involves

(a) Contact with foreign antigens
(b) Immunologic memory
(c) Slow primary response
(d) All of the above

186. Active immunity is produced by

(a) Clonal selection
(b) Clonal expansion
(c) Both (a) and (b)
(d) All of these

187. Cells involved in adaptive immunity or acquired immunity or specific defence include

(a) T cells
(b) B cells
(c) Antigen presenting cells
(d) All of these

188. Plasma cells are secreted by

(a) T cells (b) B cells
(c) Antigen presenting cells (d) Macrophages

189. The characteristics of passive immunity include

(a) Immediate relief (b) No immunologic memory
(c) Resistance for a short period only (d) All of these

190. Immunologic memory is provided by

(a) B cells (b) T cells
(c) Both (a) and (b) (d) Phagocytes

191. Humoral immunity is mediated by

(a) B cells (b) Macrophages
(c) Both (a) and (b) (d) Phagocytes

192. Humoral immunity is also called as

(a) Antibody mediated immunity
(b) Non-specific immune response
(c) Antigen mediated immunity
(d) All of these

193. B cell has receptor on its surface which is

(a) Monomeric IgM (b) Dimeric IgM
(c) Monomeric IgG (d) B cell receptor

194. B cells upon activation by antigens

(a) Undergo clonal expansion followed by clonal selection
(b) Divides continuously
(c) Undergo clonal selection followed by clonal expansion
(d) Secrete antibodies

195. B cells differentiates to form

(a) Plasma cells (b) Effector cells
(c) Plasma cells and memory B cells (d) None of these

196. Which of the following statement is incorrect regarding plasma cells

(a) Plasma cells are the effector cells
(b) Plasma cells secretes antibodies
(c) The precursor of plasma cell is B cell
(d) Plasma cell has surface receptors

197. Origin and maturation of B cells takes place at

(a) Spleen
(b) Thymus
(c) Bone marrow
(d) Lymph nodes

198. The function of memory B cell is

(a) Antibody production
(b) Immunologic memory
(c) Regulated antibody production
(d) None of these

199. B cells are

(a) Lymphocytes which are short lived
(b) Lymphocytes which are long lived
(c) Lymphocytes involved in non-specific defence
(d) None of these

200. Generally antibodies produced against a pathogen is

(a) Monoclonal
(b) Homogenous
(c) Polyclonal
(d) All of same specificity

201. Antibodies produced by plasma cells are

(a) Specific
(b) Produced against the epitope that triggered B cell activation
(c) Both (a) and (b)
(d) Diverse

202. Antibodies clear out antigens by

(a) Neutralization
(b) Precipitation
(c) Agglutination
(d) All of these

203. Antibodies are

(a) Opsonins
(b) Lipoproteins
(c) Serum phagocytes
(d) None of these

204. Any substance that promotes phagocytosis of antigens by binding to them are called as

(a) Opsonins
(b) Phagocytes
(c) Macrophages
(d) Interleukins

205. The phenomenon of selective proliferation of B cells in response to their interaction with the antigen is called

(a) Clonal expansion
(b) Monoclonal selection
(c) Clonal proliferation
(d) Clonal selection

206. Complement system

(a) Consists of 20 serum proteins

(b) Serum proteins acts as biological cascade

(c) Both (a) and (b)

(d) Are set of antibodies

207. Complement system is involved in

(a) Specific defence
(b) Non-specific defence
(c) Both (a) and (b)
(d) None of these

208. Which of the following statements are true regarding complement activation

(a) Lysis of pathogen, tumor cells and allografts

(b) Production of mediators that attracts neutrophils to the site of inflammation

(c) Opsonization

(d) All of these

209. Classical pathway of complement system is activated by

(a) Antibody-antigen complexes
(b) Antigen
(c) Antigenic peptides
(d) Antigens bound to MHC

210. Alternate pathway of complement system is activated by

(a) Antibody-antigen complexes
(b) Antigen
(c) Microorganisms or its toxins
(d) Antigens bound to MHC

211. Classical pathway of complement system is involved in

(a) Specific defence
(b) Adaptive immunity
(c) Both a and b
(d) Non-specific defence

212. Alternate pathway of complement system is involved in

(a) Non-specific defence
(b) Innate immunity
(c) Both (a) and (b)
(d) Adaptive immunity

213. Which of the following is the central molecule in complement pathway

(a) C1
(b) C2
(c) C3b
(d) C5

214. Cell lysis in complement pathway is initiated by

(a) Membrane destruction complex

(b) Membrane degradation complex

(c) Membrane attacking complex

(d) Membrane lysis complex

215. MAC is

(a) C5b6789 complex

(b) C5b5678 complex

(c) C5b5789 complex

(d) Protein polysaccharide complex

216. Which of the following is required for C1 activation

(a) Ca (b) Mg

(c) Mn (d) Zn

217. Which of the following is the most potent anaphylatoxin

(a) C3a (b) C4a

(c) C5a (d) C1

218. In alternate pathway

(a) Factor b is involved (b) Factor d is involved

(c) Both (a) and (b) (d) Only factor f is involved

219. Biological role of complement system include

(a) Cytolysis and chemotaxis

(b) Opsonisation

(c) Anaphylotoxin and enhanced antibody production

(d) All of these

220. Body's own cells are protected from membrane attack complex by a surface glycoprotein called

(a) MHC (b) DAF

(c) TCR (d) BCR

Answers

1	(b)	22	(d)	43	(c)	64	(c)
2	(a)	23	(c)	44	(a)	65	(c)
3	(c)	24	(c)	45	(d)	66	(d)
4	(c)	25	(c)	46	(b)	67	(c)
5	(a)	26	(c)	47	(d)	68	(b)
6	(b)	27	(a)	48	(d)	69	(a)
7	(b)	28	(a)	49	(d)	70	(c)
8	(a)	29	(d)	50	(d)	71	(c)
9	(b)	30	(d)	51	(c)	72	(d)
10	(d)	31	(a)	52	(a)	73	(a)
11	(b)	32	(d)	53	(d)	74	(a)
12	(c)	33	(d)	54	(d)	75	(d)
13	(d)	34	(a)	55	(d)	76	(d)
14	(a)	35	(c)	56	(d)	77	(d)
15	(a)	36	(a)	57	(c)	78	(a)
16	(b)	37	(c)	58	(a)	79	(c)
17	(b)	38	(d)	59	(d)	80	(a)
18	(a)	39	(c)	60	(c)	81	(b)
19	(b)	40	(d)	61	(a)	82	(c)
20	(a)	41	(a)	62	(a)	83	(c)
21	(a)	42	(a)	63	(a)	84	(a)

85	(d)	119	(b)	153	(b)	187	(d)
86	(c)	120	(c)	154	(a)	188	(b)
87	(d)	121	(b)	155	(b)	189	(d)
88	(b)	122	(a)	156	(d)	190	(c)
89	(d)	123	(b)	157	(b)	191	(a)
90	(c)	124	(b)	158	(c)	192	(a)
91	(d)	125	(c)	159	(b)	193	(a)
92	(a)	126	(d)	160	(b)	194	(c)
93	(c)	127	(d)	161	(c)	195	(c)
94	(c)	128	(a)	162	(d)	196	(d)
95	(d)	129	(d)	163	(d)	197	(c)
96	(d)	130	(d)	164	(b)	198	(b)
97	(b)	131	(a)	165	(d)	199	(a)
98	(b)	132	(c)	166	(d)	200	(c)
99	(b)	133	(d)	167	(c)	201	(c)
100	(a)	134	(a)	168	(c)	202	(d)
101	(c)	135	(d)	169	(a)	203	(a)
102	(c)	136	(c)	170	(c)	204	(a)
103	(a)	137	(c)	171	(d)	205	(d)
104	(a)	138	(d)	172	(c)	206	(c)
105	(a)	139	(a)	173	(c)	207	(c)
106	(a)	140	(c)	174	(c)	208	(d)
107	(a)	141	(c)	175	(b)	209	(a)
108	(d)	142	(c)	176	(d)	210	(c)
109	(b)	143	(c)	177	(d)	211	(c)
110	(c)	144	(c)	178	(a)	212	(c)
111	(a)	145	(a)	179	(c)	213	(c)
112	(c)	146	(a)	180	(a)	214	(c)
113	(a)	147	(c)	181	(b)	215	(a)
114	(d)	148	(c)	182	(c)	216	(a)
115	(c)	149	(d)	183	(c)	217	(c)
116	(a)	150	(b)	184	(a)	218	(c)
117	(c)	151	(b)	185	(d)	219	(d)
118	(a)	152	(a)	186	(c)	220	(b)

Chapter 35
Genomics–I

1. **In the case of double stranded DNA, which of the following base ratios is always equal to one**
   (a) A+T/C+G
   (b) A+G/C+T
   (c) C/G
   (d) C+T/A+C
2. **Nucleic acids are polymers of**
   (a) Nucleosides
   (b) Phosphorylated nucleosides
   (c) Glycosides
   (d) Peptides
3. **The unique feature/s of RNA, which differs it from DNA is**
   (a) Presence of uracil
   (b) Presence of ribose sugar
   (c) Both (a) and (b)
   (d) Presence of deoxyribose sugar
4. **Full form of CTAB**
   (a) Cetyltris aluminium bromide
   (b) Cesium tri ammonium boron
   (c) Carbon titarium ammonium boron
   (d) Cetyl tri methyl ammonium bromide
5. **A 10 per cent solution would be**
   (a) 10g in 1000ml of water
   (b) 10mg in 10ml of water
   (c) 10g in 100ml of water
   (d) 10 moles in 1 L
6. **Why is Ethidium Bromide used in preparation of gel**
   (a) To give gel colour
   (b) Help in visualizing DNA
   (c) For elimination of RNA
   (d) For DNA foot movement
7. **What is the full form of PCR and RFLP**
   (a) Polymerase chain reaction and restriction fragment length polymorphism
   (b) Polyacrylamide continuous reaction and recurring fusion line parent

(c) Polyacrylic combustion reaction and readymade fragment lines parents
(d) Polymerase chain reaction and restriction fragment length reaction

8. **Why blue dye is added to samples before loading them on gel**
(a) To give some catalytic action (b) To increase speed of DNA
(c) To make DNA heavy (d) For good appearance

9. **For microsatellite markers, which will be preferable gel**
(a) Agarose (b) PAGE
(c) SDA PAGE (d) Gelatin

10. **Separatin of molecular marker in gel is according to**
(a) Size (b) Charge
(c) Mass (d) Applied voltage/current

11. **What is the magnitude of amplification products on expects after "n" cycles of PCR**
(a) 3^n (b) 4^n
(c) 2^n (d) 6^n

12. **What do you mean by Tm**
(a) Melting temperature (b) Thymedine
(c) Metaphor temperature (d) Tranmembrane

13. **Which of the following markers show co-dominant inheritance?**
(a) RAPD (b) AFLP
(c) ISSR (d) SSR

14. **Function of isopropanol?**
(a) To precipitate protein (b) To extract DNA
(c) To give washing to DNA (d) To precipitate DNA

15. **CTAB is used in DNA extraction**
(a) As chelating agent (b) As washing solution
(c) To trap DNA (d) To trap proteins

16. **Which of the following markers is hybridization based?**
(a) RFLP (b) RAPD
(c) AFLP (d) STS

17. **Which of following is most useful in breeding programme?**
(a) Marker (b) Linked marker
(c) Mapped marker (d) Tightly linked marker

18. Which computer program would be useful for identification of a linked marker to trait?

(a) Microsoft Excel

(b) A sequence alignment program

(c) Mapmaker

(d) Agrobase

19. Ratio expected for co-dominant marker is in F_2 population is

(a) 1:2:1 (b) 1:2

(c) 3:1 (d) 1:1

20. Expected segregation ratio of the markers is NIL population irrespective of the nature of marker is

(a) 1:2:1 (b) 1:2

(c) 3:1 (d) 1:1

21. TILLING stands for

(a) Targeting Induced Local Lesions in Genome

(b) Traversing Inherited Local Lesions in Genome

(c) Trapping Induced Local Lesions in Genome

(d) Targeting Inherited Local Lesions in Genome

22. A system is polymorphic when its most common stage has

(a) A frequency of less than 0.95 (b) A frequency of less than 0.96

(c) A frequency of more than 0.95 (d) A frequency of more than 0.96

23. What are the parameters for supporting genetic diversity analysis during data interpretation?

(a) PIC (b) Number of alleles

(c) Per cent Polymorphism (d) All of the above

24. The graphical method used in diversity analysis is

(a) UPGMA based clustering (b) PCA

(c) Winboot analysis (d) All of the above

25. The method used for calculating heterozygosity in molecular markers based diversity analysis is

(a) PIC (b) Number of alleles

(c) Per cent Polymorphism (d) All of the above

26. Which fragment of chromosome was sequenced by India during international collaboration of Rice genome sequencing?

(a) 10S (b) 11S

(c) 10L (d) 11L

27. Which fragment of chromosome will be sequenced by India during international wheat genome sequence consortium?

(a) 1A (b) 2A
(c) 4A (d) 6A

28. Why should the chemicals used for Mol Bio work be free from exo/ endonucleases?

(a) To avoid contamination
(b) Their presence may degrade DNA
(c) Their presence may improve DNA quality
(d) To avoid hindrance in chemical reaction

29. Why is mineral oil added to top of the reaction mixture during PCR amplification in PCR

(a) To provide ions (b) To enhance amplification
(c) To avoid evaporation of the reaction (d) To increase reaction volume

30. Which enzyme is commonly used in PCR amplification?

(a) Hind III (b) Eco R 1
(c) Taq DNA polymerase (d) RNA polymerase

31. What is lyophilization?

(a) Freeze Drying (b) Melting
(c) Heating (d) Cooling of any gel

32. Specific gravity of HCl is

(a) 1.18 (b) 1.84
(c) 2.00 (d) None of above

33. Why is molecular size marker ladder loaded on gel?

(a) To provide primer
(b) To help in smooth running of the gel
(c) To compare the moleucar size of bands
(d) To see the weight of RNA and primer

34. Which of the following maker is mostly used for DNA fingerprinting these days?

(a) RFLP (b) SCAR
(c) SSR (d) STS

35. What is full form of EST's?

(a) Expression of Sigma Tags
(b) Experiment of Secale and Triticum

(c) Expressed Sequence Tags
(d) Expression of Sequences and Tools

36. MAS stands for

(a) Marker and Susceptibility (b) Mass and Size Ratio
(c) Morphological and Statistical Analysis (d) Marker Assisted Selection

37. What are cDNAs?

(a) Complementary DNA synthesized from mRNA templates
(b) Copied DNA from DNA templates
(c) Combined DNA from mRNA's
(d) Cellular DNA

38. What is the function of urea in PAGE?

(a) Catalyst (b) A binder
(c) A denaturating agent (d) As polymerizing agent

39. Which type of population is not ideal for genetic mapping?

(a) NIL (b) F2
(c) DH (d) RIL

40. What are marker systems used for high throughput genotyping?

(a) SNP (b) SRAP
(c) DArT (d) All of above

Answers

1	(a)	11	(c)	21	(a)	31	(a)
2	(b)	12	(a)	22	(a)	32	(a)
3	(c)	13	(d)	23	(d)	33	(c)
4	(d)	14	(d)	24	(d)	34	(c)
5	(c)	15	(b)	25	(a)	35	(c)
6	(b)	16	(a)	26	(c)	36	(d)
7	(a)	17	(d)	27	(b)	37	(a)
8	(c)	18	(c)	28	(b)	38	(c)
9	(b)	19	(a)	29	(c)	39	(b)
10	(a)	20	(d)	30	(c)	40	(d)

Chapter 36
Genomics–II

1. **Positional cloning efforts benefit from the human genome project because it has already identified**
   (a) Numerous useful DNA markers
   (b) The function of every human gene
   (c) The function of every human protein
   (d) The sequences of all normal and mutant alleles

2. **The first step in the positional cloning of a disease gene is to**
   (a) Identify a cDNA encoding the gene product
   (b) Map the location of a human disease gene
   (c) Clone (or copy) the gene
   (d) Identify the protein's amino acid sequence to isolate the gene

3. **DNA sequencing can reveal**
   (a) Mutations that do not alter phenotype
   (b) Mutations that do not alter genotype
   (c) Which tissues will express a gene
   (d) How many genes a person has

4. **One surprise from comparative genome projects is that**
   (a) All species examined so far have the same genes
   (b) We do not know the function of a great many genes
   (c) Small organisms can have large genomes
   (d) Large organisms can have small genomes

5. **Which genetic map is derived from restriction length polymorphisms (RFLPs) and is used to distinguish genes tens of kb apart?**
   (a) Cytogenetic map (b) Linkage map
   (c) Physical map (d) Sequence map

6. ***Mycoplasma genitalium* is the smallest microorganism known to be able to reproduce.**
   (a) True (b) False
   (c) Both may be (d) None of these

7. **According to the genomic analysis of *Mycoplasma genitalium*, what are the minimal number of genes required for life?**
   (a) 48,000 (b) 480
   (c) 265 - 350 (d) 300 Mb

8. **Which of these would be considered the simplest organism with a nucleus?**
   (a) *Saccharomyces cerevisiae* (b) *Caenorhabditis elegans*
   (c) *Drosophila melanogaster* (d) *Physcomitrella patens*

9. **Which of these is the scientific name for the fruit fly?**
   (a) *Saccharomyces cerevisiae* (b) *Caenorhabditis elegans*
   (c) *Drosophila melanogaster* (d) *Physcomitrella patens*

10. **To identify genes that are actively expressed, researchers isolate**
    (a) DNA (b) Protein
    (c) MRNA (d) CDNA

11. **cDNA is copied from _______.**
    (a) DNA (b) Protein
    (c) mRNA (d) A pictogram

12. **Expressed sequence tags (ESTs) allow researchers to identify**
    (a) Genes that encode proteins (b) Microsatellites
    (c) Ribosomal RNA genes (d) Introns

13. **Genes that are highly conserved are**
    (a) Found in a wide range of species
    (b) Repeated many times in a genome
    (c) Found in humans only
    (d) Found in a narrow range of closely related species

14. **Which of the following techniques sequences single-stranded DNA pieces on tiny beads in a water-oil mixture?**
    (a) Sanger method
    (b) Expressed sequence tag technology
    (c) C.454 sequencing
    (d) None of these

15. The size of the human genome is about ______ times larger than that of *H. influenzae.*

(a) 10 (b) 20 million

(c) 3,000 (d) 1,500

16. Who was the first person to propose sequencing of the *E. Coli* genome?

(a) Jacques Monod (b) Francis Crick

(c) Robert Sinsheimer (d) Craig Ventner

17. Sequencing shows that humans share the greatest genomic similarities with which of these?

(a) Yeast (b) Nematode worm

(c) Fruit fly (d) Chimpanzee

18. The term genome only refers to protein encoding DNA sequences.

(a) True (b) False

19. Positional cloning uses pedigree data and linkage mapping to locate a gene on a chromosome and then clone it.

(a) True (b) False

20. Positional cloning led to the discovery of genes that cause

(a) Duchene muscular dystrophy (b) Cystic fibrosis

(c) Huntington disease (d) All of these

21. Who is credited with coining the term genomics?

(a) H. Winkler (b) Patrick Brown

(c) Francis Collins (d) T. H. Roderick

22. Who is credited with first using the term genome?

(a) H. Winkler (b) Patrick Brown

(c) Francis Collins (d) James Kent

23. The 454 sequencing method can potentially sequence 20 million bases in about four and a half hours.

(a) True (b) False

24. Some people feared the human genome project would take funds away from research on AIDS and cancer.

(a) True (b) False

25. Who is credited with developing the sequencing procedure that generates a series of DNA fragments differing in length by one end base?

(a) H. Winkler (b) Frederick Sanger

(c) Francis Collins (d) James Kent

26. Who was the first director of the human genome project?

(a) James Watson (b) Francis Crick

(c) Jacques Monod (d) Craig Ventner

27. Use of expressed sequence tags (ESTs) greatly increased the amount of time it took to locate disease causing genes.

(a) True (b) False

28. Which of these require cDNA?

(a) Expressed sequence tags (ESTs) (b) The Sanger method

(c) 454 sequencing (d) Two of the above

29. The most detailed sequence information would be obtained using

(a) Expressed sequence tags (ESTs) (b) DNA microarrays

(c) 454 sequencing (d) TIGR

30. Which of these can be used to analyze the whole genome at once?

(a) Expressed sequence tags (ESTs) (b) DNA microarrays

(c) 454 sequencing (d) TIGR

31. Researchers used _______ to orient and overlap sequence data to create complete sequence maps of entire chromosomes.

(a) Sequence tagged sites (STSs) (b) DNA microarrays

(c) Fluorescent single-molecule detection (d) TIGR

32. Comparative genomics studies only protein encoding DNA sequences.

(a) True (b) False

33. _______ was the first organism to have its entire genome sequenced.

(a) The fruit fly (b) *E. coli*

(c) *Homo sapiens* (d) *Haemophilus influenzae*

34. Which of these would support the hypothesis that a disease is caused by a certain mutation?

(a) Finding the mutant gene expressed in cells affected by the disease using ESTs

(b) Finding the mutant gene expressed in the genome of affected patients using DNA microarrays

(c) Finding the mutant gene in animals affected by the disease using comparative genomics

(d) All of these

35. Knowing the complete human genome sequence will have practical applications in

(a) Health care (b) Forensics
(c) Anthropology (d) All of these

36. Which of the following represents the most reduced form of carbon?

(a) R-CH_3 (b) R-COOH
(c) R-CHO (d) R-CH_2OH

37. The *Km* (Michaelis constant) of an enzyme for a substrate is defined operationally as

(a) Half the substrate concentration at which the reaction rate is maximal
(b) The substrate concentration at which the reaction rate is half maximal
(c) The dissociation constant of the enzymesubstrate complex
(d) The dissociation constant of the enzymeproduct complex

38. Which of the following types of molecules is always found in virions?

(a) Lipid (b) Protein
(c) Carbohydrate (d) DNA

39. If the genetic code consisted of four bases per codon rather than three, the maximum number of unique amino acids that could be encoded would be

(a) 16 (b) 64
(c) 128 (d) 256

40. Eukaryotic cells with DNA damage often cease progression through the cell cycle until the damage is repaired. This type of control over the cell cycle is referred to as

(a) Proteosome control (b) Damage control
(c) Checkpoint control (d) Anticyclin control

41. Particular RNAs that are important for development are located in distinct regions of the *Drosophila* embryo. This is most directly demonstrated by using

(a) Western blotting (b) Northern blotting
(c) *In situ* hybridization (d) *In vitro* translation

42. A microarray is a large collection of specific DNA oligonucleotides spotted in a defined pattern on a microscope slide. What is the most useful experiment that can be done with such a tool?

(a) Predicting the presence of specific metabolites in a cell
(b) Comparing newly synthesized nuclear RNA with cytoplasmic RNA to locate introns

(c) Comparing RNA produced under two different physiological conditions to understand patterns of gene expression

(d) Comparing proteins produced under two different physiological conditions to understand their function

43. All of the following are proteins within the core nucleosome particle EXCEPT

(a) H1 (b) H2A

(c) H2B (d) H3

44. The KDEL sequence, found on luminal proteins of the ER, is responsible for

(a) Translocation of proteins into the ER lumen

(b) Insertion of proteins into the membrane of the ER

(c) Retrieval of ER luminal proteins from the Golgi

(d) Recognition by signal peptidase of the signal sequence

45. Cyclins are proteins involved in regulation of

(a) Cell-cycle protein kinases

(b) Circadian rhythms

(c) Synthesis of cAMP

(d) Membrane circulation via exocytosis and endocytosis

46. In a cell glycogen degradation is due to

(a) Phagocytosis of invading bacteria (b) Elevated phosphatase level

(c) Loss of acidity of lysosome in a cell (d) No major effect

47. Methylation at restriction sites in Bacterial genomes is prevented

(a) By its own endonucleases

(b) Immune mechanism

(c) Nuclease resistant genome

(d) Are not much effective on bacterial genome

48. The function of macrophages is to

(a) Enzyme Secretion (b) Engulf Cell organelles

(c) Engulf Foreign Material (d) Kills Invading Bacteria

49. The difference which distinguish prokaryotic cell from eukaryotic is

(a) ER (b) Mesosome

(c) Nuclear Membrane (d) Plasma membrane

50. Extra nuclear genetic material is found

(a) Ribosome (b) ER

(c) Chloroplast (d) Centriole

51. The acrosome of the sperm is formed from the

(a) Mitochondria
(b) Centrosome
(c) Lysomome
(d) Golgi bodies

52. Which process occur in recombination

(a) Mitosis
(b) Interphase
(c) Holiday junction
(d) DNA Repair

53. A C3 mustard plant was grown at 300 ppm of CO_2 in 14 h light and 10 h dark cycles, it was transferred to 1000 ppm CO_2. This will lead to (other environmental parameters remaining identical)

(a) Increased photosynthesis
(b) Decreased Photosynthesis
(c) Increase in Respiration
(d) No Change

54. Presence of AIDS virus cannot be detected by

(a) ELISA
(b) Western blotting
(c) Northern Blot
(d) Assay of full-length ds DNA

55. Which part of translational modification of proteins does not occur in lumen of ER

(a) Glycosylation
(b) Ubiquitnation
(c) Conformation folding and formation of quaternary structure
(d) Formation of Disulphide bonds

56. Freshly broken chromosome ends are sticky and tend to fuse, however ends of intact chromosomes are stable. Their stability is due to presence of

(a) Centromeres
(b) Telomeres
(c) Special membrane around chromosomes
(d) Kinetochores

57. Plant cell wall is generally made up of

(a) Cellulose and pectin
(b) Cellulose
(c) Chitin
(d) Murin

58. Which one of the following is correct for structure of cell wall of fungi and Bacteria?

(a) Both have glycopeptide
(b) Both are made up of N-acetylglucasamine
(c) Both are made up of murin
(d) Both are made up of chitin

59. Nucleus is absent in

(a) Sieve tube
(b) Cambium
(c) Phloem parenchyma
(d) None of these

60. Among the following which is true cell according cell theory

(a) Virus
(b) Monerans
(c) Protestans
(d) Bacteria

61. The characteristic property of metabolically active cell is

(a) Low nucleo-cytoplasmic ratio
(b) High nucleo-cytoplasmic ratio
(c) High volume to surface area ratio
(d) Small nucleus

62. Plasma membrane the functional as well as structural role is played by

(a) Proteins
(b) Lipids
(c) Cholesterol
(d) Oligosaccharides

63. Lipid nature of plasma membrane can be destroyed by

(a) Hexane
(b) Benzene
(c) Chloroform
(d) NaOH

64. The plasma membrane of intestine is highly folded into microvilli. The main function of Microvilli is

(a) To Secrete digestive enzymes
(b) To help in blood circulation
(c) To increase its absorptive surface
(d) For ageing of worn out cells

65. The structure formed where two adjacent membrane are thickened with disc shaped adhesive material in between and tonofibrils radiating out from adhesive region is

(a) Gap junction
(b) Tight junctions
(c) Desmosomes
(d) Plasmodesmata

66. The outer part of cytoplasm is usually termed as

(a) Plasmasol
(b) Plasmagel
(c) Nucleoplasm
(d) Protoplasm

67. Endoplasmic reticulum originates from

(a) Nuclues
(b) Nucleulous
(c) Golgi Complex
(d) Plasma membrane

68. The endoplasmic reticulum which constitute 50 per cent of cell is absent in

(a) Ova
(b) Embryonic cells
(c) Mature erythrocytes
(d) All of the above

69. Ribosome are attached to endoplasmic reticulum through glycoprotein known as Ribophorin I and II. The Subunit of ribosome which get attached to ER is

(a) P site (b) A site

(c) Large subunit (d) Small subunit

70. How you can separate Gram + ve bacteria from Gram –ve bacteria

(a) Presence of Techoic Acid (b) Absence of periplasmic Space

(c) Exotoxin Produced (d) All of the above

71. Lysosomes are polymorphous organelles enclosed by a single membrane. They contain vast array of hydrolytic enzymes which can digest any foreign material except

(a) Cellulose (b) Starch

(c) Glycogen (d) Lipids

72. Spectrin of erythrocytes and cytochrome c of mitochondria, which can be easily dissociated by high ionic strength and metal ion chelating agent are example of

(a) Extrinsic Protein (b) Intrinsic protein

(c) Tunnel Protein (d) Cytoplasmic Protein

73. Fats, Sterol and detoxification are found abundant in

(a) Adipose cells (b) Muscle cells

(c) Liver cells (d) All of above

74. RER is found abundantly in goblet cells, pancreatic cells and liver cells is mainly engaged in

(a) Glycosylation of protein

(b) Folding and Secondary Structure formation

(c) Production of Secretory and cytosolic protein

(d) Production and Excretion of protein

75. Microsomes are not found in cell in natural condition. They are

(a) Present only in certain bacteria

(b) Broken pieces of ER during centrifugation

(c) Broken pieces of golgi during centrifugation

(d) Present in certain fungi

76. Among the following which is not present in smaller subunit of ribosome

(a) Peptidyl transferase (b) Binding site for t RNA

(c) A Site (d) P site

77. Polyribosome are seen in

(a) Bacteria
(b) Fungi
(c) Angiosperms
(d) Mammals

78. r-RNA originates from

(a) Nucleus
(b) Nucleolous
(c) Cytoplasm
(d) ER

79. Which organelle is presenting zone of exclusion and have definite polarity

(a) Golgi
(b) ER
(c) Nucleus
(d) Ribosome

80. Lysosomes are abundant in

(a) WBC and osteoblasts
(b) RBC and Spleen
(c) Liver and Spleen
(d) WBC and Spleen

81. Lysosome membrane is strengthened by cortisol, cortisone, antihistamine, heparin, chloroquinone and cholesterol but becomes fragile

(a) Low bile salts and energy radiations
(b) In absence of oxygen
(c) Low Vitamin A and E
(d) Low Progestrone and estrogen

82. Fruit rotting can be checked by slowing down the action of enzyme polygalactouronose of the organelle

(a) Golgi
(b) Lysosomes
(c) Glyoxysome
(d) Peroxisome

83. In prokaryotes where the mitochondria is absent, the site of oxidative phosphorylation and electron transport chain including dehydrogenases is

(a) Mesosomes
(b) Endosomes
(c) Plasma membrane
(d) Microsomes

84. Water soluble phycobillin pigment occur in

(a) BGA and Green algae
(b) BGA and Red algae
(c) Green algae and Red algae
(d) Green algae and Brown algae

85. Photosynthetic pigments are located in membrane on specific areas called as

(a) Oxysomes
(b) Quantosomes
(c) Photosystem
(d) Antenna molecules

86. Microtubules are 25 nm thick, 15nm core formed of 13 helically arranged protofilaments made up of

(a) A tubulin (b) B-tubulin
(c) Myosin (d) Both a and b

87. Intermediate filaments are made up of

(a) Non-contractile proteins (b) B-tubulin
(c) Myosin (d) Actin

88. In hexose monophosphate shunt, the CO_2 molecules evolved is

(a) Same as in glycolysis (b) Less then glycolysis
(c) More then glycolysis (d) Much lesser then glycolysis

89. The electron donor during nitrogen fixation is

(a) Water (b) Ferrocynide
(c) Ferodoxin (d) CO_2

90. The chromatin is made up of repitative units known

(a) Chromosomes (b) Chromonemata
(c) Nucleosomes (d) Nucleotides

91. Exocytosis and endocytosis is absent in

(a) Amoeba (b) Euglena
(c) Mycoplasma (d) Algae

92. Cytochrome oxidase and cytochrome c deficiency in mitochondria causes

(a) Menke's disease
(b) Kearns-says syndrome and Menke's disease
(c) Kearns-says syndrome
(d) Leber's optic neuropathy

93. Photophosophorylation occurs in

(a) Plastids
(b) Mitochondria
(c) Cytoplasm
(d) Cell membrane
(e) Increased chlorophyll oxidation and necrosis

94. Which of the following is correct with regard to aneuploidy?

(a) Inversion (b) 2n + 1
(c) All aneuploid individuals die before birth (d) 4n

95. If a fragment of a chromosome breaks off and then reattaches to the original chromosome but in the reverse direction, the resulting chromosomal abnormality is called

(a) A deletion.
(b) An inversion.
(c) A translocation.
(d) A nondisjunction.

96. Why are individuals with an extra chromosome 21, which causes Down syndrome, more numerous than individuals with an extra chromosome 3 or chromosome 16?

(a) There are probably more genes on chromosome 21 than on the others.
(b) Chromosome 21 is a sex chromosome and 3 and 16 are not.
(c) Down syndrome is not more common, just more serious.
(d) Extra copies of the other chromosomes are probably fatal.

97. Humans have 23 pairs of chromosomes, while our closest relatives, chimpanzees, have 24. Chromosome studies indicate that at some point early in human evolution, two chromosomes simultaneously broke into a large portion and a small portion. The large parts combined to form a large chromosome, and the small parts combined to form a much smaller chromosome (which was subsequently lost). This important chromosomal change could best be described as

(a) Nondisjunction followed by deletion
(b) Translocation followed by deletion
(c) Duplication followed by deletion
(d) Translocation followed by inversion

98. Each cell in an individual with Down syndrome contains ____ chromosomes.

(a) 3
(b) 22
(c) 24
(d) 47

99. Disorders involving unusual numbers of sex chromosomes show that maleness is caused by the

(a) Presence of an X chromosome
(b) Presence of a Y chromosome
(c) Absence of an X chromosome
(d) Absence of a Y chromosome

100. A particular allele can have different effects if it was inherited from a male rather than a female. This phenomenon is known as

(a) Extranuclear inheritance
(b) Aneuploidy
(c) Sex-linkage
(d) Genome imprinting

101. Human mitochondria

(a) Are inherited as an X-linked trait
(b) Are all inherited from the father
(c) Have linear DNA
(d) Are all inherited from the mother

102. Both chloroplasts and mitochondria

(a) Are found within the nucleus
(b) Have linear DNA
(c) Carry extranuclear genes
(d) Are inherited from both parents

103. Damaged DNA is excised by

(a) Restriction enzymes
(b) Helicase
(c) Primase
(d) DNA polymerase

104. Unlike prokaryotic DNA replication, eukaryotic DNA replication

(a) Is completed by DNA polymerase
(b) Cannot be completed by DNA polymerase
(c) Is semiconservative
(d) Has a multiple origin

105. Which of the following is an example of a hydrophobic material?

(a) Paper
(b) Sugar
(c) Pasta
(d) Wax

106. We can be sure that a mole of table sugar and a mole of vitamin C are equal in their

(a) Weight in daltons
(b) Number of molecules
(c) Volume
(d) Number of atoms

107. Among the following which is longest cell

(a) Hemp
(b) Ramie
(c) Jute
(d) Nerve fibre

108. The middle lamella of plant cells is made up of calcium magnesium pectate. Pectic Acid is polymer of

(a) A-1,4 D-Glucose
(b) B-1,6-D Glucose
(c) A-1,4 D-Galactouronic acid
(d) B-1,4 D-Galactouronic acid

109. Acid precipitation has lowered the pH of a particular lake to 4.0. What is the hydrogen ion concentration of the lake

(a) 10^{-4} M
(b) 4.0 M
(c) 10^{-10} M
(d) 10^{4} M

110. The percentage amount of Integral protein of plasma membrane is

(a) 40 per cent
(b) 50 per cent
(c) 60 per cent
(d) 70 per cent

111. Oligosaccharide are usely attached to extrinsic phase of plasma membrane by

(a) Proteins
(b) Lipids
(c) Both (a) and (b)
(d) Not specific

112. Maximum number of enzymes in a eukaryotic cell is present inside

(a) Cytosol
(b) Mitocondria
(c) Lysosome
(d) ER

113. Which of the following term includes all others in the list?

(a) Monosaccharide
(b) Carbohydrate
(c) Disaccharide
(d) Starch

114. The structural level of a protein least affected by a disruption in hydrogen bond is the

(a) Secondary level
(b) Tertiary level
(c) Primary level
(d) Quaternary level

115. To convert a nucleoside to a nucleotide, it would be necessary to:

(a) Remove the pentose from the nucleoside
(b) Add phosphate to the nucleoside
(c) Replace purine with pyrimidine
(d) Replace ribose with deoxyribose

116. Choose the pair of terms that correctly completes this sentence

Nucleotides are to __________ as __________ are to proteins.

(a) Amino acids; polypeptides
(b) Genes; enzymes
(c) Nucleic acids; amino acids
(d) Polymers, polypeptides

117. Post translation modification of secretary proteins occurs in

(a) RER
(b) SER
(c) Mitocondria
(d) Nucleus

118. Most cells cannot harness heat in order to perform work because

(a) Heat is not a form of energy
(b) Cells do not have much heat; they are relatively cool
(c) Heat denatures enzymes
(d) Temperature is usually uniform throughout a cell

119. Choose the pair of terms that correctly completes this sentence; Catabolism is to anabolism as _________ is to _________

(a) Exergonic; spontaneous (b) Free energy; entropy

(c) Exergonic; endergonic (d) Work; energy

120. According to the first law of thermodynamics

(a) Matter can be neither created nor destroyed.

(b) All processes increase the order of the universe.

(c) Systems rich in energy are intrinsically stable

(d) Energy is conserved in all processes

121. How you can separate Gram + ve bacteria from Gram –ve bacteria

(a) Presence of Techoic Acid (b) Absence of periplasmic Space

(c) Exotoxin Produced (d) All of the above

122. The main Phagocytotic cell in immune response is

(a) Neutrophils (b) Basophils

(c) Monocytes (d) Lymphocytes

123. The phagocytes are attracted toward microorganisms by

(a) Chemotaxis (b) Rheotaxis

(c) Diapedesis (d) Thogmotaxis

124. The cell wall of microorganisms is coated with certain plasma protein promoting the attachment of microbe to phagocytes, only then they can be phagocytosised. The coat protein are called as

(a) Globins (b) Opsonins

(c) Ovulbumins (d) Phagosonins

125. After the damage of body tissues, blood vessel is dilated where damage has occurred, due to which permeability of blood vessel also increases. Vasodilation is caused by

(a) Histamine (b) Kinin

(c) Prostaglandin (d) All of above

126. The process of sneezing of phagocytes between the endothelial cells of blood vessels and reaching to damaged area is known as

(a) Margination (b) Metastasis

(c) Diapedesis (d) Angiobiosis

127. In humans interferon is produced by leucocytes, fibroblasts in connective tissue and lymphocytes and are termed as a-IFN, b-IFN and g-INF resp. The interferons are

(a) Antibacterial proteins (b) Antiviral Protein

(c) Anti cancerous protein (d) Anticancer protein

128. During embryonic stage of human B-lymphocytes are produced in

(a) Bone marrow (b) Spleen

(c) Liver (d) Bursa

129. Haptens are

(a) Immunogenic antigen

(b) Non Immunogenic Antigen

(c) High molecular weight non immunogenic antigen

(d) Low molecular weight immunogenic antigen

130. Lysosomes are polymorphous organelles containing vast array of hydrolytic enzymes which can digest any foreign material only at pH

(a) 5 (b) 6

(c) 9 (d) 7

131. Number of antigen functional binding site in human Immunoglobin-M are

(a) 2 (b) 5

(c) 10 (d) 20

132. Number of amino acids in light and heavy chain of typical immunoglobin are respectively

(a) 110, 220 (b) 220, 440

(c) 440, 880 (d) 880, 1760

133. Among the following which is not essential property of immunoglobin

(a) Memory (b) Specificity

(c) Diversity (d) Reactivity

134. Spectrin of erythrocytes and cytochrome c of mitochondria, which can be easily dissociated by high ionic strength and metal ion chelating agent are example of

(a) Extrinsic Protein (b) Intrinsic protein

(c) Tunnel Protein (d) Cytoplasmic Protein

135. Polyclonal antibodies are

(a) Clones against single antigen by many B-cells

(b) Clones against single antigen by single B-cells

(c) Clones against many antigen by single B-cells

(d) Clones against many antigen by many B-cells

136. Lymphokines that recruit the macrophages for Phagocytosis are secreted by

(a) T-cells (b) B-cells

(c) Complement system (d) MHC

137. Liposomes are

(a) Lipid filled bags
(b) Artificial membranes
(c) Liver Fat bodies
(d) Eukaryotic organelle

138. Which among the following act as bridge between cell mediated and humoral immunity

(a) T-cytoxic cells
(b) T-suppressor cells
(c) B-cells
(d) T-helper cells

139. In humans cell recognition molecules are

(a) HLA
(b) B-cells
(c) T-Cells
(d) Immunoglobins

140. Cancers cell are monoclonal, are characterized by uncontrolled growth, invasion of other tissues and dissemination to other tissues. The phenomenon of invasion to other tissues is termed as

(a) Angiobiogenesis
(b) Metastasis
(c) Diapedesis
(d) Transformation

141. A major protease secreted by cancer cells acts on plasminogen and converts it into plasmin. Plasmin is proteolytic enzyme that dissolves blood clots and also removes exposed protein groups at cell surface. If the plasminogen is removed from the medium, then

(a) The morphology of cancer cells returns to normal
(b) The cancer cell will show more exponential growth
(c) Cancer cell will die
(d) No change will be seen

142. One of the major higher molecular weight glycoprotein component which can be Easily isolated from normal cultured fibroblast by mild treatment of urea, also occur at "foot prints" that moving culture cells leaves, is totally absent in cancerous cell is

(a) Fibronectin
(b) Albumin
(c) Ferritin
(d) Transferin

143. The sex determination in drossophila is based on

(a) X-Chromosome
(b) Y chromosome
(c) Autosome
(d) Both (a) and (c)

144. Environmental control of sex determination is seen in

(a) Melandrium
(b) Drosophila
(c) Bonelia
(d) *Apes indica*

145. Protein folding is mainly driven by all of the following except

(a) Hydrophobic interactions
(b) Hydrogen bonds
(c) Covalent bonds
(d) Electrostatic attractions

146. How many Barr bodies would be present in the WBC of an individual with 49 XXXYY paratype

(a) 1
(b) 3
(c) 2
(d) 5

147. An open reading frame is one that has

(a) No start and stop codon
(b) A start and stop codon
(c) No start but stop codon
(d) A start but no stop codon

148. When the human genome draft sequence was released, which was least expected

(a) The large amount of repetitive DNA
(b) The size of total genome
(c) The size of individual chromosomes
(d) The small number of protein coding genes

149. In Sanger's Method of DNA sequencing, the growing DNA chains are terminated because

(a) DNA polymerase is not very processive
(b) A radioactive nucleotide is incorporated
(c) The substrates become limitation
(d) A phosphodiester bond can not be made

150. A recessive mutation is that

(a) Not expressed
(b) Expressed only when heterozygous
(c) Expressed only when homozygous or hemizygous
(d) Eliminated by natural selection

151. Catalytic antibodies function as enzymes on the principle of

(a) Enzymatic conversion of antibodies
(b) Stabilizing transition state analogue of substrates
(c) Antigen antibody affinity
(d) Monoclonal antibodies with chemical

152. In a Sephadex gel filteration column, a mixture of albumin, lysozyme and thymidine was loaded. In what sequence these will be eluted from the column-

(a) Albumin > Lysozyme > Thymidine

(b) Lysozyme > Thymidine > Albumin

(c) Thymidine > Albumin > Lysozyme

(d) Thymidine > Lysozyme > Albumin

153. Animal viruses cannot be seen under phase contrast microscope because

(a) They do not have a defined morphology

(b) They are too small to be seen under microscope

(c) They do not have any envelop that make them transparent under microscope

(d) Since they have no color, they are not visible

154. You have homogenized plant tissue and would like to separate chloroplast from nuclei. Which of the following methods would be most suitable

(a) PAGE

(b) Equilibrium density gradient centrifugation on CsCl gradients.

(c) Differential centrifugation using sucrose gradients.

(d) Gel filtration.

155. Which is not antibacterial antibiotic

(a) Tetracycline (b) Streptomycin

(c) Nystanin (d) Nalidixic acid

156. Degradation of RNA by RNaseA is an example of

(a) Covalent catalysis (b) Acid- base catalysis

(c) Electrostatic catalysis (d) Nucleic acid catalysis

157. Dehydrogenase enzymes of hexose mono phosphate shunt pathway are

(a) NAD specific (b) NADP specific

(c) FAD specific (d) TPP specific

158. Which of the following biochemical Rx is most commonly utilized by living cells to propagate intracellular signals?

(a) Acylation (b) Phosphorylation

(c) Methylation (d) Decarboxylation

159. Suppression mutation results in restoration of wild type phenotype. The suppression of mutant phenotype is usually brought about

(a) By misreading of mutant codon and incorporation of a correct amino acid

(b) By insertion of anather copy of gene

(c) By revertion of mutation to wild type

(d) Any deletion of mutant gene

160. A mouse in which one particular gene has been replaced by its inactivated form generated in vitro is called

(a) Transgenic mouse (b) Nude mouse

(c) Knock out mouse (d) Mutant mouse

161. Which is not a signal transducting molecule

(a) G protein coupled receptor (b) MAP kinase

(c) Protein kinase C (d) Insulin

162. Fibronectin is a protein found in

(a) RER (b) Extracellular matrix

(c) SER (d) Nuclear membrane

163. After translation proteins are modified in-

(a) Golgi apparatus (b) Lysosome

(c) Centrosome (d) Ribosome

164. In AIDS the primary problem is

(a) B cells are not functional

(b) Natural killer cells kill autologous cells

(c) Macrophages are not functional

(d) T helper are not functional

165. Which one of the following group of proteins will be most conserved among different organisms

(a) Metabolism (b) Transcription

(c) Translation (d) Cell signalling

166. The following are samples of repetitive elements that are found in a typical eukaryotic genome

(a) R-RNA (b) T-RNA

(c) SINES and LINES (d) Microsatellite

167. The ascending order in terms of number of repeats

(a) ABCD (b) DCBA

(c) CBAD (d) ADBC

168. Which sequence are best to evaluate the phylogeny of closely related mammals

(a) Coding sequences (b) Ribosomal proteins

(c) SINES and LINES (d) Centromeric and telomeric sequences

169. Leber hereditary optic neuropathy is an inherited condition what causes a loss of central vision resulting from a mutation in mitochondrial DNA. What is the probability of the children of a man with mutations in two genes and a woman with normal mitochondrial DNA inheriting this disorder as carriers?

(a) 0 per cent
(b) 100 per cent
(c) 50 per cent
(d) 66.67 per cent

170. A contig from the genome sequence of *Plasmodium falciparum*, with a single start codon when translated, was found to have high similarity with the enzyme dihydrofolate reductase and thymidylate synthase. Which of following statement is correct

(a) It contains domains present in both proteins, but neither in two enzymes
(b) It is single bi-functional protein
(c) Both the protein share a common domain
(d) The protein is unrelated to both the enzymes. There is a problem with the similarity search program used for the study

171. The consensus sequence of 5′ and 3′ splice junctions in eukaryotic m-RNA contains

(a) GU-GA
(b) GU-AG
(c) AG-GU
(d) CG-AG

172. Small cytoplasmic RNA (Sc-RNA) in eukaryotic cell

(a) Splice primary transcript
(b) Direct primary transcript
(c) Direct protein Traffic
(d) Transport amino acids

173. mRNA can be isolated by passing cell lysate through a column of oligo (dT)-Cellulose. The method is example of

(a) Partition chromatography
(b) Ion-exchange chromatography
(c) Affinity chromatography
(d) Adsorption chromatography

174. Which of the following is most commonly involved in globular shape of protein in aqueous solutions

(a) Hydrogen bonds
(b) Disulphide bonds
(c) Salt bridges
(d) Hydrophobic interactions

175. How many different gametes can be formed by an organism with genotype AaBbCCddEe ?

(a) 8
(b) 16
(c) 32
(d) 64

176. In many situations it has been found that the nucleotide sequences of two highly homologous proteins are different. It may be due to use of-

(a) Different amino acids

(b) Non-overlapping genes

(c) Different strands of DNA for encoding gene

(d) Synonymous codons due to degeneracy

177. DNA binding protein that prevents transcription are

(a) Activators (b) Operators

(c) Repressors (d) Silencers

178. The pollen tube discharges its content in

(a) The egg (b) One of synergid

(c) The central cell (d) Antipodal Cell

179. The spindle fibres in a mitotic cell are composed of

(a) Chromatin (b) Actin

(c) Nucleoprotein (d) Tubulin

180. In heterozygous cell the gene of recessive allele

(a) Is always turned off

(b) May be expressed but product is quickly degraded

(c) May be expressed without measurable effect

(d) Is deleted

181. The first step in the initiation of protein synthesis requires

(a) The 30 S ribosomal subunit (b) ATP

(c) The ribosomal A site (d) Translational factor Tu

182. House keeping genes are

(a) Inducible genes

(b) Expressed only in tumour cells

(c) Expressed in all cells

(d) Do not express at all

183. Reduction of chromosome number occurs in

(a) Mitotic anaphase

(b) Anaphase –I of meiosis

(c) Anaphase-II of meiosis

(d) Mitotic as well as meiotic anaphases

184. If the molecular mass of amino acid is 150 dalton, the molecular weight of its tripeptide will be

(a) 450
(b) 486
(c) 504
(d) 414

185. If the number of heterozygous pairs involved in a particular cross is three, the phenotype ratio obtained in their F2 generation will be

(a) 9:3:3:1
(b) 27:9:9:9:6:6:3:3:1
(c) 27:9:9:9:3:3:3:1
(d) 1:2:1:2:4:2:1:2:1

186. Rheumatoid arthritis is a/an

(a) Immunodeficiency disease
(b) Sexually transmitted disease
(c) Insect born disease
(d) Autoimmune disease

187. A linkage group corresponds to a

(a) Chromosome
(b) Set of independently assorting genes
(c) Set of independently segregating alleles
(d) Set of non complementing alleles

188. Which of the following restriction enzymes produces blunt end DNA fragments

(a) EcoR I
(b) EcoR II
(c) EcoR V
(d) Bam H1

189. Who discovered that DNA is the genetic material

(a) Arthur Kornberg
(b) James Watson
(c) Ostawald avery
(d) Severo Ochoa

190. Which of the common bases (A,C,G,T) if DNA has no oxygen in its structure

(a) Thymine
(b) Adenine
(c) Cytosine
(d) Guanine

191. What is main damaging effect of UV radiations on DNA

(a) Depurination
(b) Formation of thymine dimmers
(c) Single strand break
(d) Double strand break

192. If parents have AB and O blood group, their offspring could be of

(a) O group only
(b) A and B group
(c) A, B, O group
(d) A, B, O and AB

193. Similar set of regulatory genes control development in Arabidopsis, Drosophila and mice. These genes are called

(a) Homologous genes (b) Heterologous

(c) Homeotic (d) Orthologous

194. TATA box and Pribnow box are components of

(a) Operators (b) Promoters

(c) Enhancers (d) Activators

195. Lampbrush chromosomes occur through

(a) Diplotene of meiosis (b) Prophase of mitosis

(c) Interphase (d) Metaphase of meiosis

196. Which of the following is not associated with cell cycle

(a) Cyclins (b) Myosins

(c) CDK (d) DNA polymerases

197. Segregation of alleles takes place during the following stage of meiotic division

(a) Metaphase I (b) Anaphase I

(c) Diplotene (d) Anaphase II

198. A single crossing over between two homologous chromosomes involves

(a) Two chromatids

(b) Three chromatids

(c) Four chromatids

(d) The centromere of the chromosomes

199. Haploids are considered better genetic stock because they

(a) Are healthier then diploids

(b) Require only half of the nutrients

(c) Easy to culture

(d) Form homozygous individual on doubling

200. A yellow round seeded pea plant is crossed with green and wrinkled pea plant and the F1 of this are back crossed to the homozygous recessive parents. The progeny will appear

(a) 9:3:3:1 (b) 12:3:3:1

(c) 3:3:3:1 (d) 1:1:1:1

201. Which of the following is the approximately size of human genome

(a) 4×10^6 bp (b) 1×10^{10} bp

(c) 3×10^9 bp (d) 5×10^{65} bp

202. Which of the following type of DNA is the most conserved amongst organisms

(a) Mitochondrial DNA
(b) Chloroplast DNA
(c) RDNA
(d) DNA that codes for t-DNA

203. Which of the following is incorrect regarding Chargaff's rule

(a) [A] = [T]
(b) [G] =[C]
(c) [A] + [T] = [G] + [C]
(d) [A]+ [G] = [T] + [C]

204. If total concentration of A=T is 56 per cent. What will be concentration of cytosine in genome

(a) 56
(b) 23
(c) 44
(d) 22

205. In the B form of DNA, the paired bases are planar, parallel to one another and they are

(a) Parallel to long axis of double helix
(b) Perpendicular to long axis of double helix
(c) Inclined to long axis
(d) Inverted in respect to long axis

206. Among the Following staggered cut is obtained by

(a) Alu I
(b) Rsa I
(c) Pst I
(d) Pvu (II)

207. Which one is the essential feature of restriction sites cut by restriction endonucleases II

(a) Palindromic
(b) Within recognisation site
(c) Always methylated
(d) All the above

208. The genomic size of E. coli is 4.6 X 10 6 bp, if a 6 base pair cutter is utilized to obtain restriction fragments, then what will be total number of fragments obtained

(a) 1.12×10^3
(b) 7.66×10^5
(c) 25×10^4
(d) 3.83×10^3

209. Tm (Melting temperature) would be maximum for

(a) *Saricina lutea*
(b) *E. coli*
(c) *Drosophila*
(d) Human

210. Natural absorption of UV by DNA is due to nucleotide base pairs which increase on denaturation. They absorb maximum amount of UV wavelength of

(a) 200 nm
(b) 260 nm
(c) 280 nm
(d) 355 nm

211. For Nucleic acid hybridization which condition is not essential

(a) The salt conc. must be high (>25 M)
(b) Primers
(c) High temperature, under control
(d) Complementary strands

212. Genetic variations, in form of multiple alleles of many genes, exist in most of natural population. Such genetic differences between individuals are called DNA polymorphism. Such a DNA polymorphism is used as

(a) DNA markers
(b) DNA probes
(c) C-DNA
(d) Heteroduplex DNA

213. The best DNA markers utilized to differentiate different human individuals (to establish paternity and divergence) are

(a) Single Nucleotide Polymorphism
(b) Rest Fragment Length Polymorphism
(c) Random Amplified Polymorphic DNA
(d) Simple tandem repeats polymorphism

214. Which chemical group are present at the extreme 3′ ends of single polynucleotide strand

(a) Phosphate group
(b) Hydroxyl group
(c) Oxo group
(d) CH_2OH

215. The template DNA strand utilized for DNA replication is

(a) 5'-3' direction
(b) 3'-5 direction
(c) Random
(d) In both direction

216. The enzyme coded by allele IA transferase which adds Nacetyl glucasmine and blood group is designated as A, similarly IB encodes transferase which adds galactose to precursor sugar, similarly IO encodes transferase which adds

(a) No sugar
(b) N-acetyl glucasamine
(c) Galactose
(d) Both galactose and N acetyl glucasmine

217. If two recessive mutations are alleles of different genes, then F1 progeny are wild type, this is due to

(a) Incomplete dominance
(b) Complementation
(c) Supplementation
(d) Co-dominance

218. Sexual differentiation in Drosophila is controlled by gene called sex lethal (sxl). The genes sensing the number of x chromosomes are called as

(a) Supernumery genes
(b) Denominator genes
(c) Numerator genes
(d) Sex sensing genes

219. What would be sex of Drosophila with chromosome complement 3A + XXYY

(a) Male (b) Female

(c) Inetersex (d) Metamale

220. Eukaryotic gene regulation occurs at the level of:

(a) Posttranslational control (b) Transcriptional control

(c) Genomic control (d) All of the above

221. Ubiquitin binds to ________ residues, therefore targeting proteins for degradation by ________.

(a) Lysine, proteasomes (b) Arginine, lysosomes

(c) Arginine, proteasomes (d) Lysine, lysosomes

222. Protein phosphoryation, dephosphorylation and proteolytic cleavage are examples of

(a) Posttranslational control (b) Transcriptional control

(c) Translational control (d) Control of RNA processing

223. Steroid hormone receptors are involved in

(a) Control of RNA processing (b) Posttranslational control

(c) Transcriptional control (d) Genomic control

224. Which of the following is NOT an example of genomic control of gene regulation?

(a) Alternative RNA splicing (b) DNA rearrangement

(c) Gene deletion (d) Gene amplification

225. Which of the following is true of homeotic genes?

(a) The homeodomain functions in binding to DNA

(b) They serve as an example of transcriptional gene control

(c) All homeotic genes contain a 180-bp segment called a homeobox

(d) All of the above are correct

226. ________ is an allosteric protein that is inactive until it binds to ________, thus activating transcription.

(a) RNA polymerase, cAMP (b) CRP, ATP

(c) CRP, cAMP (d) RNA polymerase, ATP

227. The trp leader sequence contains a control region that is sensitive to tryptophan levels such that it determines whether transcription will continue to completion. The effect of this control element in the trp operon in E. coli is known as

(a) Gene amplification (b) RNA splicing

(c) Attenuation (d) Repression

228. Histone structure can be altered by

(a) DNA rearrangement
(b) Acetylation
(c) Sigma factors
(d) Methylation

229. Which of the following is true of heatshock genes?

(a) They are only found in prokaryotes
(b) They encode for proteins such as progesterone and estrogen
(c) They are only found in eukaryotes
(d) They are known to respond to stressful conditions

230. A gene is

(a) The same thing as a chromosome
(b) The information for making a polypeptide
(c) Made of RNA
(d) Made by a ribosome

231. In Eukaryotes, DNA packing affects gene expression by

(a) Controlling access to DNA.
(b) Positioning related structural genes near each other
(c) Protecting DNA from mutations
(d) Enhancing recombination of genes

232. Dioxin, produced as a byproduct of various industrial chemical processes, is suspected of causing cancer and birth defects in animals and humans. It apparently acts by entering cells and binding to proteins, altering the pattern of gene expression. The proteins affected by dioxin are probably

(a) Water-soluble proteins
(b) DNA polymerase
(c) Transcription factors
(d) Enhancers

233. In humans, the hormone testosterone enters cells and binds to specific proteins, which in turn bind to specific sites on the cells DNA. These proteins probably act to

(a) Help RNA polymerase transcribe certain genes
(b) Alter the pattern of DNA splicing
(c) Inhibit transcription.
(d) Unwind the DNA for gene transcription

234. It is possible for a cell to make proteins that last for months; hemoglobin in red blood cells is a good example. However, many proteins are not this longlasting. They may be degraded in days or even hours. Why do cells make proteins with such short lifetimes if it is possible to make them last longer?

(a) Most proteins are used only once
(b) Most cells in the body live only a few days

(c) Cells lack the raw materials to make most of the proteins they need
(d) Only cancer cells, which can keep dividing, contain long-lasting proteins

235. The genes that malfunction in cancer normally
(a) Control RNA transcription
(b) Are responsible for sex determination
(c) Code for enzymes that repair damaged DNA
(d) Are not present in most body cells

236. Which of the following are arranged in the correct order by size, from largest to smallest?
(a) Chromosome-gene-codon-nucleotide
(b) Nucleotide-chromosome-gene-codon
(c) Codon-chromosome-gene-nucleotide
(d) Gene-chromosome-codon-nucleotide

237. Imagine an error occurring during DNA replication in a cell, so that where there is supposed to be a T in one of the genes there is instead a G. What effect will this probably have on the cell?
(a) Each of its kinds of protein will contain an incorrect amino acid
(b) An amino acid will be missing from each of its kinds of protein
(c) One of its kinds of protein might contain an incorrect amino acid
(d) The amino acid sequence of one of its kinds of protein will be completely changed

238. What is the role of promoter in DNA sequence
(a) Transfer RNA acts to translate the message to RNA polymerase
(b) The ribosome directs it to the correct portion of the DNA molecule
(c) It looks for the AUG start codon
(d) RNA polymerase recognize and start transcribing a gene into m RNA

239. All your cells contain proto-oncogenes, which can change into cancercausing genes. Why do cells possess such potential time bombs?
(a) Viruses infect cells with proto-oncogenes
(b) Proto-oncogenes are genetic junk and have no known function
(c) Proto-oncogenes are unavoidable environmental carcinogens
(d) Cells produce proto-oncogenes as a by-product of mitosis

240. In Eukaryotes, which of the following mechanisms of gene regulation operates after mRNA transcription but before translation of mRNA into protein?
(a) mRNA splicing and editing (b) DNA packing
(c) Repressors and activators (d) Protein degradation

241. A cell biologist found that two different proteins with largely different structures were translated from two different mRNAs. These mRNAs, however, were transcribed from the same gene in the cell nucleus. Which mechanism below could best account for this?

(a) Different systems of DNA unpacking could result in two different mRNAs

(b) A mutation might have altered the gene

(c) Exons from the same gene could be spliced in different ways to make different mRNAs

(d) The two mRNAs could be transcribed from different operons

242. A particular ________ carry the information for making a particular polypeptide, but ________ can be used to make any polypeptide.

(a) Gene and ribosome; a tRNA and an mRNA

(b) Gene and mRNA ; a ribosome and a tRNA

(c) Ribosome and mRNA; a gene and a tRNA

(d) Gene and tRNA ; a ribosome and an mRNA

243. Which of the following processes occurs in the cytoplasm of a eukaryotic cell?

(a) DNA replication

(b) Translation

(c) Transcription

(d) DNA replication and translation

244. The nucleotide sequence of a DNA codon is GTA. A messenger RNA molecule with a complementary codon is transcribed from the DNA. In the process of protein synthesis, a transfer RNA pairs with the mRNA codon. What is the nucleotide sequence of the tRNA anticodon?

(a) CAT (b) GUA

(c) CAU (d) GTA

245. The nucleotide sequence of a DNA codon is ACT. A messenger RNA molecule with a complementary codon is transcribed from the DNA. In the process of protein synthesis, a transfer RNA pairs with the mRNA codon. What is the nucleotide sequence of the tRNA anticodon?

(a) TGA (b) UGA

(c) TGU (d) ACU

246. During the process of translation (polypeptide synthesis), ________ matches an mRNA codon with the proper amino acid.

(a) A ribosome (b) DNA polymerase

(c) ATP (d) Transfer RNA

247. A sequence of pictures of polypeptide synthesis shows a ribosome holding two transfer RNAs. One tRNA has a polypeptide chain attached to it; the other tRNA has a single amino acid attached to it. What does the next picture show?

(a) The polypeptide chain moves over and bonds to the single amino acid

(b) The amino acid moves over and bonds to the polypeptide chain

(c) The tRNA with the polypeptide chain leaves the ribosome

(d) A third tRNA with an amino acid joins the pair on the ribosome

248. A geneticist found that a particular mutation had no effect on the polypeptide coded by a gene. This mutation probably involved

(a) Deletion of one nucleotide
(b) Alteration of the start codon
(c) Insertion of one nucleotide
(d) Substitution of one nucleotide

249. A mutagen is

(a) A gene that has been altered by a mutation

(b) Something that causes a mutation

(c) An organism that has been changed by a mutation

(d) The portion of a chromosome altered by a mutation

250. There are thought to be about __________ genes in a human cell.

(a) 30 – 100
(b) 300 – 1,000
(c) 3,000 – 10,000
(d) 30,000 – 50,000

251. Histones are

(a) Master genes that affect development

(b) Groups of genes that respond to environment

(c) Proteins around which DNA is coiled

(d) Portions of genes that are transcribed

252. During Interphase, __________ can be seen with a light microscope.

(a) Nucleosomes
(b) Introns
(c) Heterochromatin
(d) Euchromatin

253. There is about 1,000 times as much DNA in a human cell as in an *E. coli* cell, but only about 50 times as many genes. Why?

(a) A human cell has much more noncoding DNA

(b) The DNA packing is much more complex in a prokaryotic cell

(c) Most of the genes in a human cell are turned off

(d) *E. coli* are less able to respond to their environment than humans. Moreover, this response confuses cause and effect

254. The difference between tandemly repetitive and interspersed repetitive DNA is that

(a) Interspersed DNA is also referred to as satellite DNA

(b) Interspersed repetitive DNA is found throughout the genome.

(c) Most tandemly repetitive DNA are transposons

(d) Most interspersed repetitive DNA is at the telomeres

255. Multigene families arise as a result of

(a) Transformation

(b) Errors during DNA replication and recombination

(c) RNA splicing

(d) Protein degradation

256. Retrotransposons differ from other transposons in that

(a) Retrotransposons have lost the ability to move about a genome

(b) Retrotransposons are likely to be the remains of a viral infection

(c) Retrotransposons have retained the ability to move about a genome, an ability that has been lost by other transposons

(d) Retrotransposons move via an RNA transcript, whereas other transposons do not

257. Your muscle and bone cells are different because

(a) They contain different sets of genes

(b) They are differentiated

(c) They contain different operons

(d) Different genes are switched on and off in each type of cell

258. Gene expression in animals seems to be regulated largely by

(a) Controlling gene packing and unpacking

(b) Controlling the transcription of genes into mRNA

(c) Controlling the translation of mRNA into protein

(d) Selectively eliminating certain genes from the genome

259. The control of gene expression is more complex in multicellular eukaryotes than in prokaryotes because

(a) Eukaryotic cells are much smaller

(b) In a multicellular eukaryote, different cells are specialized for different functions

(c) Prokaryotes are restricted to stable environments

(d) Eukaryotes have fewer nucleotide, so each nucleotide sequence must do several jobs

260. Which of the following would be most likely to lead to cancer?

(a) Multiplication of a proto-oncogene and inactivation of a tumor-suppressor gene

(b) Hyperactivity of a proto-oncogene and activation of a tumor-suppressor gene

(c) Failure of a proto-oncogene to produce a protein and multiplication of a tumor-suppressor gene

(d) The failure of both a proto-oncogene and a tumor-suppressor gene to produce proteins

261. Your bone cells, muscle cells, and skin cells look different because

(a) Different kinds of genes are present in each kind of cell

(b) They are present in different organs

(c) Different genes are active in each kind of cell

(d) They contain different numbers of genes

262. Linkage groups are equivalent to haploid set of chromosomes, if male butterfly has 12 linkage groups, then female will have

(a) 12 (b) 11

(c) 13 (d) 6

263. Maximum possible recombination frequency is

(a) 25 per cent (b) 50 per cent

(c) 75 per cent (d) 100 per cent

264. The linkage of genes in chromosomes can be represented in form of

(a) Genetic maps (b) Linkage maps

(c) Chromosome map (d) All of these

265. Physically 1 map unit on linkage maps can be defined as length of chromosome in which, average crossover formed during 50 cells undergoing meiosis is

(a) 1 (b) 25

(c) 50 (d) 100

266. Assuming equal sex ratio, what is probability that a sib ship of four children consists entirely of boys

(a) 25 per cent (b) 12. 5 per cent

(c) 6.25 per cent (d) 3.125 per cent

267. The spindle fibres attach to each chromosome in the region technically known as

(a) Centromere (b) Centriole

(c) Kinetochoere (d) Astrals

268. Which among the following do not have DNA

(a) Kinetoplast (b) Centriole

(c) Dictyosomes (d) Chindriosomes

269. During meiosis the centromeric division takes place during

(a) Prophase I (b) Anaphase I

(c) Prophase II (d) Anaphase II

270. Which of the following cell junctions is responsible for metabolic coupling?

(a) Tight junction (b) Gap junction

(c) Adherens junction (d) Desmosome

271. Which of the following statements about repetitive DNA is NOT true?

(a) Repetitive DNA is associated with the centromeres and telomeres in higher eukaryotes

(b) Repetitive DNA is restricted to nontranscribed regions of the genome

(c) Repetitive DNA sequences are often found in tandem clusters throughout the genome

(d) Repetitive DNA was first detected because of its rapid reassociation kinetics

272. The ability of a cell to migrate on a substrate involves all of the following EXCEPT

(a) Formation and breakage of focal adhesions

(b) Assembly of an actin meshwork at the leading edge

(c) Connexin proteins

(d) Arp2/3 complex proteins

273. Allosteric inhibition of an enzyme involves which of the following?

(a) Binding of an inhibitor to a site other than the substrate binding site

(b) Binding of an inhibitor competitively to the substrate binding site

(c) Binding of an inhibitor noncompetitively to the substrate binding site

(d) Cooperative binding of substrate to an enzyme with four or more subunits

274. Which of the following represents the sequence of electron flow in the light reactions of photosynthesis in higher plants?

(a) $H_2O \rightarrow$ photosystem I $\rightarrow$ photosystem II $\rightarrow$ NADP

(b) $H_2O \rightarrow$ photosystem II $\rightarrow$ photosystem I $\rightarrow$ NADP

(c) $H_2O \rightarrow$ photosystem II $\rightarrow$ photosystem I $\rightarrow$ ATP

(d) NADPH $\rightarrow$ photosystem I $\rightarrow$ photosystem II $\rightarrow O_2$

275. The urea cycle occurs in the

(a) Mitochondrion and cytoplasm (b) Mitochondrion and lysosome
(c) Endoplasmic reticulum (d) Golgi complex

276. The glyoxylate cycle is found in plants and bacteria but not in animals. The lack of this cycle in animals results in the inability to

(a) Synthesize oxaloacetate from isocitrate
(b) Synthesize glutamate from malate
(c) Perform gluconeogenesis from amino acids
(d) Perform gluconeogenesis from fatty acids

277. Mitosis and meiosis accomplish segregation of the replicated DNA to two or more daughter cells. Which of the following is characteristic of both mitosis and meiosis?

(a) Chromosomes attach to spindle fibers composed of actin
(b) The resulting cells are diploid (2n)
(c) The resulting cells are haploid (1n)
(d) Spindle fibers attach to chromosomes at their kinetochores

278. One important mechanism for maintaining sequence identity among the many copies of a gene within a tandem array is

(a) Unequal crossing-over (b) Gene conversion
(c) Retrotransposition (d) Deletion

279. In *E. coli*, the inability of the *lac* repressor to bind an inducer would result in

(a) No substantial synthesis of -galactosidase
(b) Constitutive synthesis of -galactosidase
(c) Inducible synthesis of -galactosidase
(d) Synthesis of inactive -galactosidase

280. An RNA-dependent RNA polymerase is likely to be present in the virion of a

(a) DNA virus that multiplies in the cytoplasm
(b) DNA virus that multiplies in the nucleus
(c) Minus-strand RNA virus
(d) Plus-strand RNA virus

281. All of the following are known to be part of a signal transduction cascade EXCEP

(a) Phosphorylation of fibronectin
(b) Dissociation of the components of a heterotrimeric G-protein
(c) Enzymatic breakdown of phosphatidyl inositol bisphosphate (PIP2)
(d) Elevation of intracellular [Ca^{2+}]

282. The initial product of photosynthetic CO_2 fixation in C_3 plants is

(a) Glyceraldehyde 3-phosphate
(b) Dihydroxyacetone phosphate
(c) 3-phosphoglycerate
(d) Phosphoenolpyruvate

283. Which enzyme is activated by phosphorylation?

(a) Acetyl-CoA carboxylase
(b) Fructose-1,6-bisphosphatase
(c) Glycogen synthase
(d) Fructose-2,6-bisphosphatase

284. SNARE proteins are found in the membranes of all of the following compartments EXCEPT

(a) Mitochondria
(b) Golgi complex
(c) Early endosome
(d) Endoplasmic reticulum

285. Treatment of root tip meristem cells with the microtubule inhibitor colchicine results in all ofthe following EXCEPT

(a) Induction of polyploidy
(b) Prevention of cytokinesis
(c) Inhibition of mitotic spindle assembly
(d) Cessation of DNA replication

286. Proline disrupts -helical structure in proteins because it is

(a) An acidic amino acid
(b) An aromatic amino acid
(c) An imino acid
(d) A basic amino acid

287. Which of the following statements about retrotransposons is correct?

(a) They transpose via an RNA intermediate
(b) They contain genes for ribosomal proteins
(c) They possess a gene for RNA-dependent RNA polymerase
(d) They possess genes that encode proteins that integrate RNA into chromosomes

288. Membrane carrier proteins differ from membrane channel proteins by which of the following characteristics?

(a) Carrier proteins are glycoproteins, while channel proteins are lipoproteins.
(b) Carrier proteins transport molecules down their electrochemical gradient, while channel proteins transport molecules against their electrochemical gradient
(c) Carrier proteins can mediate active transport, while channel proteins cannot.
(d) Carrier proteins do not bind to the material transported, while channel proteins do

289. The common pathway of entry into the endoplasmic reticulum (ER) of secretory, lysosomal, and plasma membrane proteins is best explained by which of the following?

(a) Binding of their mRNAs to a special class of ribosomes attached to the ER

(b) Addition of a common sorting signal to each type of protein after completion of synthesis

(c) Addition of oligosaccharides to all three types of proteins

(d) Presence of a signal sequence that targets each type of protein to the ER during synthesis

290. A microarray is a large collection of specific DNA oligonucleotides spotted in a defined pattern on a microscope slide. What is the most useful experiment that can be done with such a tool?

(a) Predicting the presence of specific metabolites in a cell

(b) Comparing newly synthesized nuclear RNA with cytoplasmic RNA to locate introns

(c) Comparing RNA produced under two different physiological conditions to understand patterns of gene expression

(d) Comparing proteins produced under two different physiological conditions to understand their function

291. Acetyl CoA, the cytoplasmic substrate for fatty acid synthesis, is formed in mitochondria. The inner mitochondrial membrane is impermeable to acetyl CoA. Which of the following compounds is the form in which the carbon of acetyl CoA is transported to the cytoplasm?

(a) Malate (b) Acetate

(c) Citrate (d) Pyruvate

292. Which of the following groups of enzymes are unique to the Calvin cycle?

(a) Ribulose bisphosphate carboxylase, phosphoribulokinase, and sedoheptulose 1,7-bisphosphatase

(b) Ribose 5-phosphate isomerase, epimerase, and aldolase

(c) Glyceraldehyde 3-phosphate dehydrogenase, phosphofructokinase, and phosphoenolpyruvate carboxylase

(d) Phosphoglycolate phosphatase, glycerol kinase, and serine synthetase

293. The synthesis of mRNA's that encode the proteins of eukaryotic ribosomes occurs in the

(a) Cytoplasm (b) Nuclear envelope

(c) Nucleolus (d) Euchromatin

294. Which of the following best supports the endosymbiotic theory of the evolutionary origin of mitochondria?

(a) Mitochondria, chloroplasts, and prokaryotes contain electron carriers

(b) Genes for mitochondrial pyruvate dehydrogenase subunits are found in the nuclear DNA

(c) Mitochondrial and bacterial ribosomal functions are inhibited by the same antibiotics

(d) The outer mitochondrial membrane contains the protein porin

Answers

1	(a)	23	(a)	45	(a)	67	(a)
2	(b)	24	(a)	46	(c)	68	(d)
3	(a)	25	(b)	47	(a)	69	(c)
4	(b)	26	(a)	48	(c)	70	(d)
5	(c)	27	(b)	49	(c)	71	(a)
6	(a)	28	(a)	50	(c)	72	(a)
7	(c)	29	(c)	51	(d)	73	(c)
8	(a)	30	(b)	52	(c)	74	(d)
9	(c)	31	(a)	53	(a)	75	(b)
10	(c)	32	(b)	54	(d)	76	(a)
11	(c)	33	(d)	55	(b)	77	(a)
12	(a)	34	(d)	56	(b)	78	(b)
13	(a)	35	(d)	57	(a)	79	(a)
14	(c)	36	(a)	58	(b)	80	(d)
15	(d)	37	(b)	59	(a)	81	(b)
16	(b)	38	(a)	60	(d)	82	(c)
17	(d)	39	(d)	61	(b)	83	(a)
18	(b)	40	(c)	62	(a)	84	(b)
19	(a)	41	(c)	63	(b)	85	(b)
20	(d)	42	(c)	64	(c)	86	(d)
21	(d)	43	(a)	65	(c)	87	(a)
22	(a)	44	(c)	66	(b)	88	(c)

89	(c)	123	(a)	157	(c)	191	(b)
90	(c)	124	(b)	158	(c)	192	(b)
91	(c)	125	(d)	159	(a)	193	(c)
92	(b)	126	(c)	160	(c)	194	(b)
93	(a)	127	(b)	161	(d)	195	(a)
94	(b)	128	(c)	162	(b)	196	(b)
95	(b)	129	(d)	163	(a)	197	(b)
96	(d)	130	(a)	164	(d)	198	(a)
97	(b)	131	(c)	165	(a)	199	(d)
98	(d)	132	(b)	166	(c)	200	(d)
99	(b)	133	(d)	167	(a)	201	(c)
100	(d)	134	(c)	168	(b)	202	(b)
101	(d)	135	(d)	169	(a)	203	(c)
102	(c)	136	(a)	170	(b)	204	(d)
103	(a)	137	(b)	171	(b)	205	(b)
104	(d)	138	(d)	172	(d)	206	(c)
105	(a)	139	(a)	173	(c)	207	(b)
106	(b)	140	(b)	174	(d)	208	(d)
107	(a)	141	(d)	175	(b)	209	(a)
108	(d)	142	(a)	176	(d)	210	(b)
109	(a)	143	(d)	177	(c)	211	(b)
110	(d)	144	(c)	178	(b)	212	(a)
111	(c)	145	(c)	179	(d)	213	(d)
112	(b)	146	(c)	180	(b)	214	(b)
113	(c)	147	(b)	181	(a)	215	(b)
114	(c)	148	(d)	182	(c)	216	(a)
115	(b)	149	(d)	183	(b)	217	(c)
116	(c)	150	(c)	184	(d)	218	(c)
117	(a)	151	(b)	185	(c)	219	(c)
118	(d)	152	(a)	186	(d)	220	(d)
119	(c)	153	(b)	187	(a)	221	(a)
120	(d)	154	(c)	188	(d)	222	(a)
121	(d)	155	(c)	189	(c)	223	(c)
122	(a)	156	(d)	190	(b)	224	(a)

225	(d)	243	(b)	261	(c)	279	(a)
226	(c)	244	(b)	262	(a)	280	(c)
227	(c)	245	(d)	263	(b)	281	(a)
228	(b)	246	(d)	264	(d)	282	(c)
229	(d)	247	(b)	265	(c)	283	(d)
230	(b)	248	(d)	266	(c)	284	(a)
231	(a)	249	(b)	267	(c)	285	(d)
232	(c)	250	(d)	268	(c)	286	(c)
233	(a)	251	(c)	269	(d)	287	(a)
234	(b)	252	(c)	270	(b)	288	(c)
235	(c)	253	(a)	271	(b)	289	(d)
236	(a)	254	(b)	272	(d)	290	(c)
237	(c)	255	(b)	273	(a)	291	(c)
238	(d)	256	(d)	274	(b)	292	(a)
239	(b)	257	(d)	275	(a)	293	(b)
240	(a)	258	(b)	276	(d)	294	(c)
241	(c)	259	(b)	277	(d)		
242	(b)	260	(a)	278	(b)		

Chapter 37

Microbiology–I

1. **If the bacteria doubles itself in 5 minutes, what would be number of bacteria at end of 20 minutes if you start with 4 bacteria**
   (a) 64 (b) 32
   (c) 48 (d) 16

2. **The percentage of protein coding sequence in *E.coli* is**
   (a) 2 per cent (b) 0.2 per cent
   (c) 70 per cent (d) 30 per cent

3. **Among the following which is considered as the best indicator of water pollution**
   (a) *Bacillus* (b) *Clostridium*
   (c) *E. coli* (d) *Paramecium*

4. **The F+ segments of bacteria may be transferred to F- bacteria by the process of**
   (a) Conjugation (b) Transformation
   (c) Transduction (d) Fragmentation

5. **It has been observed that in bacterial colonies bacteria often secrete toxins at high population density to check the population size. This phenomenon is termed**
   (a) Population control (b) Allelopathy
   (c) Intra specific competition (d) Quorum sensing

6. **If bacterial genome and plasmid are allowed to replicate in same manner then among the following which is characteristic feature of meiosis I**
   (a) Bacteria genome will replicate faster (b) Plasmid will replicate faster
   (c) Both will replicate in same time (d) Depends on GC content

7. **A prophage is**
   (a) DNA of lysogenic phage inserted into host chromosome
   (b) Is a stage of cell cycle
   (c) Lambda phage DNA
   (d) Plasmid

8. **Bacteria propels with the help of**
   (a) Myosin (b) Actin
   (c) Cytoskeleton (d) Flagella made of flagellin

9. **In operons, if repressor binds to operator, it will lead to**
   (a) Initiation of transcription (b) Enhancement of transcription
   (c) Blocks transcription (d) Differential gene expression

10. **The glycocalyx around cell membrane can be determined by**
    (a) Iodine (b) Crystal violet
    (c) Lectins (d) Saffranin

11. **Among the following which activity is absent in bacterial DNA polymerase I**
    (a) 3′-5′ exonucleases activity (b) 5′-3′ exonucleases activity
    (c) 3′-5′ polymerase activity (d) 5′-3′ polymerase activity

12. **Transduction has been used extensively for genome mapping for bacteria, which of the following process is useful for gene mapping**
    (a) Bacterial lysis (b) Generalised transduction
    (c) Specialized transduction (d) Site specific recombination

13. ***Mycobacterium tuberculosis* causes disease by entering into host cell and not allowing the endosome to mature into**
    (a) ER (b) Lysosome
    (c) Peroxisome (d) Granulocytes

14. **Exponential growth in bacteria would be expected during**
    (a) Lag phase (b) Stationary phase
    (c) Log phase (d) Deceleration pahse

15. **Sendai virus enters host cell by**
    (a) Receptor mediated endocytosis (b) Phagocytosis
    (c) Cell fusion (d) Cell fusion

Answers

1	(a)	5	(d)	9	(c)	13	(b)
2	(c)	6	(b)	10	(c)	14	(c)
3	(c)	7	(a)	11	(c)	15	(c)
4	(a)	8	(d)	12	(b)		

Chapter 38
Microbiology–II

1. **A major difference between EHEC and EPEC is**
   (a) EHEC secretes a Shiga-like toxin and EPEC does not
   (b) EHEC possesses a type III secretion system and EPEC does not
   (c) EPEC rearranges host cell actin and EHEC does not
   (d) EPEC passes through the placenta to infect the fetus and EHEC does not

2. **The nature of the poliovirus gives for oral vaccination (satin vaccine) as part of the eradication programme is**
   (a) Heat killed virus
   (b) Live attenuated strains of all three immunological types
   (c) Small dosage of wild-type live viruses
   (d) Formalin-inactivated viruses

3. **Which of the following is true regarding anthrax?**
   (a) Anthrax is caused by a virus
   (b) Anthrax is highly contagious
   (c) Inhalation anthrax and cutaneous anthrax are caused by separate strains of *Bacillus anthracis*
   (d) Inhalation Anthrax requires infection with a large number of spores

4. **The toxins produced by bacteria**
   (a) Kill viruses
   (b) Encourage bacterial reproduction
   (c) Interfere with physiological processes in the body
   (d) All of the above

5. **Pseudomembraneous colitis is**
   (a) Precipitated by the use of certain antibiotics
   (b) Caused by a gram-positive bacterium

(c) Caused by a spore-forming bacterium
(d) All of the above

6. Both *Mycobacterium tuberculosis* and *Streptococcus pneumoniae*
(a) Are acquired by inhalation
(b) Have cell walls that contain a high content of mycolic acids
(c) Have polysaccharide capsules
(d) Stay in the lung and rarely, if ever, enter the bloodstream

7. Cholera toxin is an A-B type toxin in which the B portions bind to a receptor on a host cell and the A portion enters the cell to cause
(a) ADP ribosylation of adenylate cyclase that stops production of cAMP
(b) ADP ribosylation of a G protein that locks it into an active form that stimulates adenylate cyclase to make cAMP
(c) Cleavage of rRNA that results in disruption of ribosome function
(d) ADP ribosylation of guanylate cyclase that stimulates production of cGMP

8. Mucus helps in protecting against pathogens by
(a) Lowering the pH
(b) Facilitating the growth of normal flora
(c) Blocking access and attachment of pathogens to mucosal surfaces
(d) Sequestering Iron

9. Type III secretion systems are used to inject "effector" proteins directly into a host cell. *Salmonella* uses a type III secretion system to help the pathogen to
(a) Survive the acid pH of the stomach
(b) Secrete LT (heat labile toxin) and ST (heat stable toxin) into the lumen of the intestine
(c) Survive within macrophages
(d) Activate T cells to proliferate and secrete cytokines

10. Which of these cytokines is also known under the name cachectin?
(a) Interferon gamma (b) Interleukin 2
(c) Tumor necrosis factor (TNF) (d) None of the above

11. Which is not a major defense mechanism in the stomach?
(a) Proteolytic enzymes (b) Low pH
(c) Dense normal flora (d) All of these

12. The agent responsible for causing mad cow disease is thought to be a
(a) Fungus (b) Protozoan
(c) Prion (d) Virus

13. The "A" subunit of diphtheria toxin

(a) Binds host cell receptors found on heart cells

(b) Cause ADP ribosylation of a factor involved in protein synthesis

(c) Forms cAMP that leads to fluid accumulation

(d) Lysis macrophages with the release of cytokines

14. Coxsackie virus B3, a subgroup of enteroviruses, commonly causes

(a) Acute haemorrhagic conjunctivitis (b) Muscular dystrophy

(c) Myocarditis (d) Gastroenteritis

15. Prontosil is

(a) An effective antibacterial when used in animals

(b) An effective antibacterial when used in in-vitro cultures

(c) An effective antibacterial both in animals as well as in in-vitro cultures

(d) Not used as an antibacterial agent

16. All infections do not cause fever and all fevers are not due to infections which of the following is an example of non-infections cause of fever?

(a) Typhoid (b) Chicken pox

(c) Rheumatic disease (d) Malaria

17. Immunization with which of the following toxoid induces high titer serum antibody, but does not protect from the corresponding disease?

(a) Tetanus (b) Botulism

(c) Diphtheria (d) Shigellosis

18. Which of the following statements is not true regarding *Mycobacterium tuberculosis* and/or the disease it causes?

(a) The pathogen contains mycolic acid in its cell wall

(b) The pathogen can live inside macrophages

(c) Antibodies to the pathogen are protective

(d) None of these

19. What is common in catheters and ventilators?

(a) They bypass important defenses of the body

(b) Bacteria responsible for associated infections are usually susceptible to antibiotics

(c) They predispose patients to viral rather than bacterial infections

(d) They are used primarily in neonatal intensive care units

20. An important host defense of human beings is a dense resident microbiota associated with

(a) Lungs (b) Bladder

(c) Uterus (d) Vagina

21. Lactoferrin helps to protect against pathogens by

(a) Sequestering Iron

(b) Blocking sebum production

(c) Facilitating the growth of normal flora

(d) Lowering the pH

22. The influenza vaccine is administered each year because

(a) Mutations in the viral hemagglutinin may allow the virus to evade the immune response elicited by previous vaccines

(b) It is a polysaccharide vaccine that does not confer long-term protection

(c) The vaccine is sufficiently toxic to make it necessary to administer only a small amount at any one time

(d) None of the above

23. Which of the following disease is caused by DNA viruses?

(a) Poliomyelitis (b) Yellow fever

(c) Measles (d) Small pox

24. Which of the following is common in the disease caused by *Coryne-bacterium diphtheriae* and *Bacillus anthracis*?

(a) Both organisms are gram-positive spore formers

(b) Diphtheria toxin and edema toxin are ADP ribosylating toxins

(c) The most serious disease symptoms are the direct result of toxin action

(d) Both organisms cause skin and respiratory tract infections

25. Fatalities following influenza infection are usually due to the

(a) Dehydration

(b) Bacterial superinfection

(c) Damage to the heart muscle

(d) Formation of granulomas in the lung

26. Which of the following disease is not caused by microbial protein toxin?

(a) Botulism (b) Diphtheria

(c) Shigella dysentery (d) Tuberculosis

27. In the human disease cholera, what is it that actually ends up killing the victim?

(a) Faulty carrier proteins

(b) Dehydration and loss of nutrients

(c) Too little water in the food stream

(d) The toxin produced by the bacterium

28. Each of the 3 virulence factors of *Bacillus anthracis i.e.* the capsule, edema toxin and lethal toxin can affect the activity of

(a) B cells (b) Macrophages

(c) Ciliated epithelial cells (d) M cells

29. The nonsymbiotic bacteria which fix nitrogen live in the soil independently are

(a) *Azotobacter*

(b) *Clostridium*

(c) Considerably less important in comparison to the symbiotic bacteria

(d) All of the above

30. Nitrogen fixation by the microorganisms can be detected by adopting the approach of

(a) Demonstrating growth in a nitrogen free medium

(b) Cultivating the microorganisms in the presence of nitrogen labeled with isotropic nitrogen

(c) Measuring $^{15}N_2$ by mass spectrometer

(d) All of the above

31. Which of the following is not the biofertilisers producing bacteria?

(a) Nostoc (b) Anabaena

(c) Both (a) and (b) (d) Clostridium

32. Which of the following is capable of oxidizing sulfur to sulfates?

(a) *Thiobacillus thiooxidans* (b) *Desulfotomaculum*

(c) *Rhodospirillum* (d) *Rhodomicrobium*

33. Most soil protozoa are flagellates or amoebas, having their dominant mode of nitrogen as

(a) Ingestion of bacteria (b) Ingestion of mold

(c) Ingestion of fungi (d) All of these

34. Which of the following microorganism use H_2S as the electron donor to reduce carbon dioxide?

(a) *Chromaticum*
(b) *Chlorobium*
(c) Both (a) and (b)
(d) *Rhodomicrobium*

35. Nitrifying bacteria can not be isolated directly by the usual techniques employed to isolate hetrotrophic bacteria. The reasons may be due to

(a) Slow growth
(b) Medium growth
(c) Fast growth
(d) None of these

36. Bacteria, as a group, are responsible for

(a) Nitrogen oxidation
(b) Sulfur oxidation
(c) Nitrogen fixation
(d) All of these

37. The phenomenon of commensalism refers to a relationship between organisms in which

(a) One species of a pair benefits
(b) Both the species of a pair benefit
(c) One species of a pair is more benefited
(d) None of the above

38. The population of algae in soil is __________ that of either bacteria or fungi.

(a) Generally smaller than
(b) Generally greater than
(c) Equal to
(d) None of these

39. The transformation of nitrates to gaseous nitrogen is accomplished by microorganisms in a series of biochemical reactions. The process is known as

(a) Nitrification
(b) Denitrification
(c) Nitrogen fixation
(d) Ammonification

40. Nitrogen fixation refers to the direct conversion of atmospheric nitrogen gas into

(a) Ammonia
(b) Glucose
(c) ATP
(d) Nitrate

41. The diagnostic enzyme for denitrification is

(a) Nitrate reductase
(b) Nitrate oxidase
(c) Nitro oxidoreductase
(d) None of these

42. A heterocyst is

(a) A type of spore
(b) A terminally differentiated cell that fixes nitrogen
(c) The progenitor of cyanobacterial vegetative cells
(d) A cell that carries out oxygenic photosynthesis

43. The groups of symbiotic bacteria, which have the ability to fix nitrogen

(a) Derive their food and minerals from the legume, and in turn they supply the legume with some or all of its nitrogen

(b) Grow together for a mutual benefit is called symbiosis and so these bacteria are called symbiotic nitrogen-fixing bacteria

(c) These bacteria are from the genus, Rhizobium

(d) All of the above

44. An example of a symbiotic nitrogen fixer is

(a) *Azotobacter* (b) *Beijerinckia*

(c) *Clostridium* (d) *Rhizobium*

45. Which of the following is correct?

(a) Mycorrhizae are fungi that form a mutually beneficial (symbiotic) relationship with plant roots

(b) The fungi aid in transmitting nutrients and water to the plant roots

(c) The increased nutrient availability from mycorrhizae is thought to be due to the additional absorbing surface provided by the fungi

(d) All of the above

46. In the process of nitrogen fixation, which of the following microorganism is involved?

(a) Non symbiotic microorganisms only

(b) Symbiotic microorganisms only

(c) Non symbiotic and symbiotic microorganisms only

(d) None of the above

47. Which of the following statement is not true about composition of biogas?

(a) It is composed almost exclusively of methane and carbon dioxide

(b) It also contains with traces of H_2S, N_2, $H_2$and CO

(c) It also contains with traces of O_2 and Cl_2

(d) Both (a) and (b)

48. The physical structure of soil is improved by the accumulation of

(a) Mold mycelium (b) Minerals

(c) Water (d) All of these

49. __________ play a key role in the transformation of rock to soil.

(a) Cyanobacteia (b) Pectin decomposing bacteria

(c) Nitrifying bacteria (d) De-nitrifying bacteria

50. The groups of bacteria which have the ability to fix nitrogen from air to soil are

(a) Symbiotic (b) Nonsymbiotic
(c) Both (a) and (b) (d) None of these

51. The nitrogenase consists of

(a) Dinitrogenase (b) Dinitrogenase reductase
(c) Both (a) and (b) (d) None of these

52. The crops which are involved in nitrogen fixation are

(a) Alfalfa and clover (b) Soybean
(c) Bean and lupine (d) All of these

53. Denitrification may be distinguished as

(a) Dissimilative (b) Assimilative
(c) Both (a) and (b) (d) Blue baby syndrome

54. The conversion of molecular nitrogen into ammonia is known as

(a) Nitrification (b) Denitrification
(c) Nitrogen fixation (d) Ammonification

55. The breakdown of cattle manure in biogas is accomplished by which of the following type of bacteria?

(a) Hydrolytic (b) Transitional
(c) Methanogenic (d) All of these

56. Which of the following species of different genera of bacteria are not capable of transforming nitrate to nitrogen?

(a) *Achromobacter* (b) *Agrobacterium*
(c) *Alcaligenes* (d) None of these

57. Some microorganisms have the ability to increase the nitrogen content of soils, are called as

(a) Nitrogen fixation (b) Denitrification
(c) Nitrification (d) All of these

58. Nitrogen fixation

(a) Changes the free nitrogen (N_2) to a form usable by plants
(b) Especially changes nitrogen compounds, mostly amines such as NH_2
(c) Both (a) and (b)
(d) Fix the free nitrogen (N_2) by which it should not be usable by plants

59. For rapid decomposition by microbes, the substrate should have a C/N ratio of

(a) 10-20 (b) 20-30
(c) 30-40 (d) 60-80

60. Which are the main source of biofertilisers?

(a) Cyanobacteria (b) Bacillus
(c) Streptococcus (d) None of these

61. The organisms responsible for the characteristic musty or earth odor of a freshly plowed field is/are

(a) Nocardia (b) Streptomyces
(c) Micromonospora (d) All of these

62. Denitrification is

(a) Reduction of nitrate (NO_3^-) to nitrogen gas
(b) Reduction of nitrate to organic nitrogen compounds
(c) Both (a) and (b)
(d) Changing of atmospheric nitrogen (N_2) to nitrogen compounds

63. Degree of compost maturity can be assesed by

(a) Infrared technique (b) Germination test
(c) Both (a) and (b) (d) None of the above

64. The energy value of biogas is typically

(a) 400-700 BTU/ft^3 (b) 1,000 BTU/ft^3
(c) 1500 BTU/ft^3 (d) More than 5000 BTU/ft^3

65. The microbial ecosystem of soil includes

(a) Biotic components of soil (b) Abiotic components of soil
(c) Biotic and abiotic components of soil (d) None of the above

66. Denitrification is carried out

(a) Usually by facultative anaerobes
(b) Predominantly by *Pseudomonas* spp.
(c) Predominantly by *Bacillus* spp.
(d) All of the above

67. Which of the following soil microorganism is involved in the reduction of sulfates to H_2S?

(a) *Thiobacillus thiooxidans* (b) *Desulfotomaculum*
(c) *Rhodospirillum* (d) *Rhodomicrobium*

68. The diagnostic enzyme for nitrogen-fixing organisms is

(a) Nitrogenase (b) Nitrate reductase
(c) Nitrate oxidase (d) None of these

69. Which of the following fungi on infecting crop roots can improve their uptake of phosphorus and other nutrients?

(a) *Saccharomyces cerevisiae* (b) VA Mycorrhiza
(c) *Candida torulopsis* (d) *Aspergillus niger*

70. Syntrophism involves

(a) Exchange of nutrients between two species
(b) Exchange of nutrients among species
(c) No exchange of nutrients between two species
(d) No exchange of nutrients among species

71. Assimilative denitrification is done by

(a) Plants (b) Fungi
(c) Prokaryotes (d) All of these

72. The concept of putting microbes to help clean up the environment is called

(a) Pasteurization (b) Bioremediation
(c) Fermentation (d) Biolistics

73. Which of the following is not employed as an oxidation method?

(a) Oxidation ponds (b) Trickling filters
(c) Contact aerators (d) All of these

74. The filtering medium of trickling filters is coated with microbial flora, known as

(a) Zoological film (b) Geological film
(c) Zooglocal film (d) None of these

75. Some cyanobacteria produce potent neurotoxins that, if ingested, will kill humans. These cyanobacteria are most likely to contaminate

(a) Water rich in organic carbon wastes but poor in phosphate
(b) Water that are anoxic
(c) Water rich in phosphate wastes but poor in organic carbon
(d) None of the above

76. The biogas production process takes place at the temperature

(a) Lesser than 25°C (b) 25-40°C
(c) 45-60°C (d) All of these

77. Advanced treatment is generally used to treat waste water to

(a) Remove coarse solids

(b) Remove settleable solids

(c) Reduce BOD

(d) Remove additional objectionable substances

78. Treatment of municipal water supplies is based upon

(a) Coagulation, filtration, chlorination

(b) Chlorination, filtration, coagulation

(c) Filtration, coagulation, chlorination

(d) Coagulation, chlorination, filtration

79. What is an anaerobic digester?

(a) New diet drink

(b) Microbe that eats hazardous waste

(c) Method to convert agricultural waste into a biogas

(d) All of the above

80. The use of microbes to break down synthetic waste products such as polychlorinated biphenyls is called

(a) Bioinformatics (b) Biolistics

(c) Biotechnology (d) Bioremediation

81. Activated sludge contains large number of

(a) Bacteria (b) Yeasts and molds

(c) Protozoa (d) All of these

82. Iron bacteria can produce

(a) Slime (b) Undesirable odors and tastes

(c) Both (a) and (b) (d) Extreme acidity

83. Biomass

(a) Provides the U.S. with about 50 per cent of its energy

(b) Consists largely of wood, animal, and human waste

(c) Is unlikely to be a major source of energy globally

(d) Offers the consumer high quality energy with low environmental impact

84. Composting is one of the oldest forms of disposal of waste. It is the natural process of decomposition of organic waste that yields manure or compost. One of the following is added to the compost to get better results?

(a) Ants (b) Bugs

(c) Snakes (d) Worms

85. Which is not a form of biomass energy?

(a) Incineration of solid waste
(b) Composting to produce methane
(c) Ethanol and methanol production for auto fuel
(d) Photovoltaic production of hydrogen

86. Which of the following statement is not correct?

(a) The use of 25-40°C temperatures allows the biogas production to be more stable
(b) The use of 25-40°C temperatures does not destroy potentially harmful bacteria
(c) The use of 25-40°C temperatures destroys potentially harmful bacteria
(d) None of the above

87. Oxidation ponds are shallow ponds, generally designed at the depth of

(a) 2 to 40 feet
(b) 4 to 6 feet
(c) 1 to 3 feet
(d) 5 to 8 feet

88. Which of the following is generally not referred to the sewerage system?

(a) Sanitary sewers
(b) Storm sewers
(c) Combined sewers
(d) Solid sewers

89. The magnitude of BOD of wastewater is related to

(a) Bacterial count
(b) Amount of organic material
(c) Amount of inorganic material
(d) All of the above

90. A dense bacterial population caught in a tangled web of fibers sticking to a surface describes

(a) The membrane filter technique
(b) A biodisc
(c) A biofilm
(d) Coagulation

91. Biogas production is

(a) A temperature-dependent process
(b) An oxygen dependent process
(c) A temperature independent process
(d) None of the above

92. The acetate-utilizing methanogens are responsible for

(a) 20 per cent of methane produced in a biogas reactor
(b) 50 per cent of methane produced in a biogas reactor
(c) 70 per cent of methane produced in a biogas reactor
(d) 85 per cent of methane produced in a biogas reactor

93. Which of the following is responsible for the corrosion problem?

(a) Iron bacteria (b) Sulfur bacteria
(c) Slime forming bacteria (d) All of these

94. Water testing relies on the detection of certain indicator organisms known as

(a) Acid-fast bacteria (b) Bacteroids
(c) Coliforms (d) Dinoflagellates

95. The death of a river by environmental pollutants ultimately results from

(a) The overpopulation of algae
(b) The overabundance of toxic proteins
(c) The depletion of oxygen
(d) The buildup of sediment on the river bottom

96. The phospholipids present in cytoplasm membrane of the archaeo-bacteria is

(a) Phosphoglycerides (b) Polyisoprenoid
(c) Polyisoprenoid branched chain lipids (d) None of the above

97. The oldest eukaryotic organisms are considered to be

(a) Diplomonads like Giardia (b) Archaea
(c) Fungi (d) Animals

98. The phospholipids present in cytoplasm membrane of eubacteria is mainly

(a) Phosphoglycerides (b) Polyisoprenoid
(c) Phospholipoprotein (d) None of these

99. Which were the investigators lived at the same time?

(a) Koch and Pasteur (b) Darwin and Woese
(c) Van Leeuenhoek and Ricketts (d) Berg and Hooke

100. The unifying feature of the archaea that distinguishes them from the bacteria is

(a) Habitats which are extreme environments with regard to acidity
(b) Absence of a nuclear membrane temperature
(c) Presence of a cell wall containing a characteristic outer membrane
(d) Cytoplasmic ribosomes that are 70S

101. Mycoplasmas are different from the other prokaryotes by

(a) Presence of chitin in cell walls
(b) Presence of murrain in cell walls
(c) Presence of proteins in cell walls
(d) Absence of cell wall itself

102. Evolutionary relationships between groups of organisms are determined using which of the following type of information?

(a) Comparisons of nucleotide sequences

(b) Comparisons of biochemical pathways

(c) Comparisons of structural features

(d) All of the above

103. Which of the following is not true for eukaryotic cells?

(a) Nucleus is bounded by nuclear membrane

(b) Chromosomes contain histones

(c) Chloroplasts and mitochondria contains 70S ribosomes

(d) Gas vacuoles are present

104. Which of the following is not true for prokaryotic organism?

(a) Nucleus is not bounded by nuclear membrane

(b) Chromosomes does not contain histones

(c) 80S ribosomes are distributed in cytoplasm

(d) Cell wall contains peptidoglycan as one of the major component

105. Gram staining was introduced by

(a) Christian gram (b) Alfred Gram

(c) Robertcook (d) Louis Pasteur

106. Which of the following is considered the most unifying concept in biology?

(a) Taxonomy (b) Anatomy

(c) Genetics (d) Evolution

107. Various bacterial species can be subdivided into

(a) Subspecies (b) Biovarieties

(c) Serovarieties (d) All of these

108. Living organisms have many complex characteristics. Which one of the following is shared by non-living matter as well?

(a) Homeostasis (b) Tissues

(c) Reproduction (d) Molecules

109. A newly discovered microscopic structure is hypothesized to be a living organism. Which of the following lines of evidence would support the contention that this organism may be alive?

(a) It contains DNA (b) It is made of a single cell

(c) It utilizes energy (d) All of these

110. Mycoplasmas, rickettsiae, and chlamydiae are

(a) Types of fungi
(b) Small bacteria
(c) Species of protozoa
(d) Forms of viruses

111. Which of the following structure is absent in eukaryotic cells?

(a) Mitochondria
(b) Chloroplasts
(c) Golgi structure
(d) Mesosome

112. Who was the inventor of the Petri dish?

(a) R.J. Petri, an assistant of R. Koch
(b) A famous French cook
(c) Italian glass blower from Petri, Italy
(d) None of the above

113. Which one is not studied in microbiology?

(a) Bacteria
(b) Animal behaviour
(c) Fungi
(d) Algae

114. A characteristic of protein synthesis in both the archaea and eukarya is

(a) Transcription and translation are coupled
(b) Translation is inhibited by diphtheria toxin
(c) Proteins are synthesized from D-, rather than L-, isomers of amino acids
(d) The initiator tRNA is charged with N-formyl-methionine

115. Cell theory includes all of the following except

(a) All organisms are composed of one or more cells
(b) The cell is the most primitive form of life
(c) The cell is the structural unit of life
(d) Cells arise by division of pre-existing cells

116. The five-kingdom system of classification was set up by

(a) Louis Pasteur
(b) Robert Whittaker
(c) Robert Koch
(d) Masaki Ogata

117. The membranes of which domains are chemically the most similar?

(a) Archaea and Bacteria
(b) Bacteria and Eukarya
(c) Eukarya and Archaea
(d) Membranes of all three domains are chemically identical

118. Primary differences between cilia and flagella are

(a) Arrangement of microtubules
(b) Length and location of basal bodies
(c) How the microtubules are fused to each other
(d) Number, length and direction of force

119. All membranes of free-living organisms have phospholipid bilayers, but exception is

(a) Bacteria
(b) Fungi
(c) Archaea
(d) Protozoa

120. All of the following are features of prokaryotes except

(a) Nitrogen fixation
(b) Photosynthesis
(c) Sexual reproduction
(d) Locomotion

121. Which of the following structures is the smallest?

(a) Viriod
(b) Hydrogen atom
(c) Bacterium
(d) Mitochondrion

122. Which of the following is/are included in Kingdom *Prokaryotae*?

(a) Bacteria
(b) Protozoa
(c) Fungi
(d) All of these

123. Which of the following may account for the small size of the cells?

(a) The rate of diffusion
(b) The surface area/volume ratio
(c) The number of mRNAs that can be produced by the nucleus
(d) All of the above

124. Genetic and biochemical similarities between contemporary cyanobacteria and eukaryotic chloroplasts are accepted to mean that

(a) Eukaryotes evolved from bacteria
(b) Eukaryotes evolved from archaea
(c) Oxygenic photosynthesis first evolved in eukaryotes
(d) Cyanobacteria arose from chloroplasts which escaped from plant cells

125. Which of the following best represents the hierarchy of levels of biological classification?

(a) Phylum, kingdom, class, order, genus, species, family
(b) Kingdom, phylum, class, order, family, genus, species
(c) Kingdom, phylum, family, class, order, genus, species
(d) Class, order, kingdom, phylum, family, genus, species

126. The three domain version of life on earth is based on the

(a) Nucleic acid sequence data
(b) Morphological traits
(c) Metabolic traits
(d) Characteristics of the cell wall

127. The foundation for the germ theory of disease was set down by

(a) Robert Koch (b) Ronald Ross

(c) Louis Pasteur (d) Walter Reed

128. Most microbial structures and enzymes are composed of

(a) Lipids (b) Proteins

(c) Carbohydrates (d) Lipids and carbohydrates

129. The individual best remembered for bringing microbes to the world is

(a) Robert Hooke (b) Antony Van Leeuenhoek

(c) Robert Koch (d) Masaki Ogata

130. Micro organisms are found in which of the following kingdom of five kingdom concept (Whittaker's classification)?

(a) Monera (b) Protista

(c) Fungi (d) All of these

131. The first organism in most natural food chains is

(a) A herbivore (b) A decomposer

(c) Photosynthetic (d) Carnivorous

132. The third kingdom, protista, as suggested by E.H. Haeckel includes

(a) Bacteria (b) Algae

(c) Fungi (d) All of these

133. Eukaryotic cell organelles first emerged

(a) From a specialized lineage of cells within the kingdom Protista

(b) When prokaryotes engulfed each other and became interdependent

(c) When bacteria made their first attempts at reproduction

(d) Just before the origin of the animal and fungal kingdoms

134. Who discovered the bacteria that cause cholera?

(a) Pierre Berthelot (b) Robert Koch

(c) Louis Pasteur (d) Rudolf Virchow

135. Prokaryotic microorganism include

(a) Protozoa (b) Fungi

(c) Bacteria (d) All of these

136. All the following are basic properties of cells except

(a) Cells have nuclei and mitochondria

(b) Cells have a genetic programme and the means to use it

(c) Cells are capable of producing more of themselves

(d) Cells are able to respond to stimuli

137. Which of the following microorganisms is classified as a member of archaebacteria?

(a) Gyanobacteria (b) Methanobacteria
(c) Trichomonads (d) Mycoplasma

138. The idea of selective toxicity was first proposed by

(a) Antony van Leeuwenhoek (b) Paul Ehrlich
(c) Louis Pasteur (d) Alexander Fleming

139. Which of the following sequences has helped in identifying eukaryotes, eubacteria and archeabacterial cell types?

(a) Signature sequence (b) Signal sequence
(c) Shine-Dalgarno sequence (d) Amino acid sequence

140. Archeal cells usually do not contain peptidoglycan, rather contain pseudo-peptidoglycan which is mainly composed of

(a) N-acetylmuramic acid and L-amino acids
(b) N-acetylmuramic acid and D-amino acids
(c) N-acetyltalosaminuronic acid and D-amino acids
(d) N-acetyltalosaminuronic acid and L-amino acids

141. In the three domain system of classification, the traditional bacteria are placed in the

(a) Eukarya (b) Archaea
(c) Eubacteria (d) None of these

142. One of the reasons for the evolutionary success of the kingdom Monera is that its members are nutritionally diverse. Which of the following(s) is/are the way(s) of obtaining energy?

(a) Photoautotrophy (b) Photoheterotrophy
(c) Chemoheterotrophy (d) All of the above

143. Carl Woese and his colleague are best known for establishing

(a) The five kingdom system (b) The three domain system
(c) The prokaryote-eukaryote system (d) The plant-animal system

144. Which of the following is not found in the kingdom Monera?

(a) Organelles (b) Organized cell structure
(c) Ability to reproduce (d) Ability to use energy

145. Which of the following is the most primitive?

(a) Virus (b) Eukaryote
(c) Archaeon (d) Mitochondria

146. All the following are considered eukaryotes except

(a) Archaea (b) Fungi

(c) Protozoa (d) Humans

147. Which cell type is considered to have the oldest ancestor?

(a) *Archaea* (b) Bacteria

(c) They all share the same ancestor (d) *Eukarya*

148. What is Mycology?

(a) Study of viruses (b) Study of nucleic acid

(c) Study of bacteria (d) Study of fungi

149. Which of the following organelles contain DNA, divides and possesses some degree of autonomy?

(a) Golgi apparatus (b) Ribosome

(c) Chloroplast (d) Peroxisomes

150. All of the following individuals contributed to cell theory except

(a) Robert Hooke (b) Matthias Schleiden

(c) Theodor Schwann (d) Rudolf Virchow

151. Eukaryotic micro organisms include

(a) Protozoa (b) Fungi

(c) Algae (d) All of these

152. The binomial name of a microbe is composed of

(a) Its kingdom and genus names

(b) Its genus name and a species modifier

(c) Its family and class names

(d) Its genus and species names

153. Which of the following is a characteristic unique to the ciliates?

(a) Use of cilia as a sensory function

(b) Presence of both a macronucleus and several micronuclei

(c) Both (a) and (b)

(d) Possess a light-detecting eye spot

154. Which of the following structure is present in prokaryotic cells?

(a) Mitochondria (b) Chloroplasts

(c) Golgi structure (d) Mesosome

155. The word cell was first used by

(a) Robert Hooke
(b) Theodor Schwann
(c) Louis Pasteur
(d) Ronald Ross

156. What are Blue-Green bacteria called?

(a) *Acquaobacteria*
(b) *Cyanobacteria*
(c) *Protozoa*
(d) None of the above

157. The endosymbiosis hypothesis provides an explanation for how

(a) Eukaryotes developed from prokayotes
(b) Prokaryotes developed from eukaryotes
(c) Algae developed from protozoa
(d) Protozoa developed from algae

158. The Archaea include all of the following except

(a) Methanogens
(b) Halophiles
(c) Thermoacidophiles
(d) Cyanobacteria

159. During the carboxylation phase of the Calvin cycle, CO_2 combines with

(a) Ribulose 1,5 - bisphosphate
(b) Phosphoglyceraldehyde
(c) Pyruvic acid
(d) Oxaloacetic acid

160. Which of the following groups contain(s) many unique coenzymes, such as coenzyme M and coenzyme F_{420}?

(a) Sulfate-reducing bacteria
(b) Methanotrophs (methane-oxidizing microbes)
(c) Methanogens (methane-producing microbes)
(d) Acetogens (acetigens; acetate-producing microbes)

161. In the passive diffusion, solute molecules cross the membrane as a result of

(a) Concentration difference
(b) Pressure difference
(c) Ionic difference
(d) All of these

162. In an oxygenic photosynthesis, the green and the purple bacteria do not use which of the following one as an electron source?

(a) H_2O
(b) H_2
(c) H_2S
(d) S (elemental sulphur)

163. Radioisotopes are frequently used in the study of cells. Assume a culture of *E. coli* is grown in a culture medium containing radioactive phosphorous. At the end of 48 hours, it is expected to find the radioactive label located in

(a) Enzymes
(b) RNA
(c) Phospholipids
(d) All of these

164. Assimilatory sulfate reduction involves the nucleotide __________ during the incorporation of H_2S in the production of __________.

(a) ATP; methionine
(b) ATP; cytosine
(c) UTP; cytosine
(d) GTP; cytosine

165. The chlorophyll molecules used by eucaryotes and cyanobacteria absorb radiant energy in the __________ portion(s) of the visible spectrum.

(a) Red
(b) Green
(c) Red and blue
(d) Green and ultraviolet

166. In aerobic respiration, the terminal electron acceptor is

(a) Oxygen
(b) Nitrogen
(c) Hydrogen
(d) Nitrate

167. Which of the following statement is correct?

(a) Phosphate repression can not be eliminated by optimization of nutrient medium, deregulated medium must be used as production strains
(b) Phosphate repression can be eliminated by optimization of nutrient medium, deregulated medium must be used as production strains
(c) Phosphate repression can be eliminated by optimization of nutrient medium, regulated medium must be used as production strains
(d) Phosphate repression can not be eliminated by optimization of nutrient medium, regulated medium must be used as production strains

168. The acquisition energy by glucose fermentation requires

(a) Substrate-level phosphorylation
(b) Electron transport of electrons from NADH
(c) Long-chain fatty acid oxidation
(d) The enzyme formic-hydrogen lyase

169. High energy transfer compounds are capable of

(a) Accepting large amounts of free energy
(b) Transferring large amounts of free energy
(c) Measuring free energy
(d) None of the above

170. Dolichol phosphate is

(a) A complex lipid involved in docking vesicles with the plasma membrane
(b) The anchor on which sugars assemble before transfer to proteins
(c) A chaperone used in protein folding
(d) A product of phospholipase C activation

171. The reactions of the cell that are carried out for capturing energy are called

(a) Catabolism
(b) Metabolism
(c) Anabolism
(d) Activation energy

172. In establishing proton gradient for chemiosmotic ATP generation by aerobic respiration the terminal electron acceptor is

(a) Nitrate
(b) Oxygen
(c) Sulfate
(d) CO_2

173. If ΔG of a chemical reaction is positive in value and k_{eq} is less than 1 then the chemical reaction will

(a) Proceed in reverse direction
(b) Proceeed in forward direction
(c) Not take place in any of the direction
(d) None of these

174. The reaction, where small precursor molecules are assembled into larger organic molecules is referred as

(a) Anabolism
(b) Catabolism
(c) Metabolism
(d) Any of these

175. Which of the following nucleoside diphosphates is used most often in carbohydrate anabolism?

(a) Uridine diphosphate
(b) Adenosine diphosphate
(c) Guanine diphosphate
(d) Thymine diphosphate

176. DAHP synthetase catalyzes the condensation of

(a) Erythrose-4-phosphate
(b) Phosphoenol pyruvate
(c) Both (a) and (b)
(d) Phenylalanine

177. Phosphate is considered to restrict the induction of

(a) Primary metabolites
(b) Secondary metabolites
(c) Both (a) and (b)
(d) None of these

178. Free energy change (ΔG) of a reaction is referred as the amount of energy

(a) Liberated during reaction
(b) Taken up during reaction
(c) Liberated or taken up during reaction
(d) None of these

179. Which of the following does not produce oxygen as a product of photosynthesis?

(a) Oak trees
(b) Purple sulfur bacteria
(c) Cyanobacteria
(d) Phytoplankton

180. When acetate is the sole source of carbon for some microorganisms, the cycle which is used, is called

(a) Pentose phosphate pathway
(b) Glycolyic pathway
(c) Glyoxylate pathway
(d) Oxaloacetate pathway

181. Hexose monophosphate pathway is also known as

(a) Phosphogluconate pathway
(b) Oxaloacetate pathway
(c) Malate pathway
(d) Fumerate pathway

182. If radioactive bicarbonate was supplied to bacterial cells, which were actively synthesizing fatty acids, it is expected to find the bulk of the radioactivity in

(a) Cellular bicarbonate
(b) The fatty acids
(c) The cytoplasmic membrane
(d) Nucleic acids

183. Standard free energy change (ΔG) can be expressed as

(a) $\Delta G° = -RTlnk_{eq}$
(b) $\Delta G° = RTlnk_{eq}$
(c) $\Delta G° = R/Tlnk_{eq}$
(d) $\Delta G° = -RT/lnk_{eq}$

184. The glyoxylate cycle is used by some microorganisms when __________ is the sole carbon source.

(a) Acetate
(b) Nitrate
(c) Carbon dioxide
(d) All of these

185. The role of bacteriophyll in an oxygenic photosynthesis is to

(a) Reduce ferridoxin directly
(b) Reduce NADP directly
(c) Use light energy to energize an electron
(d) Transfer electrons to an intermediate in the sulfide oxidation pathway

186. TCA cycle functions in

(a) Catabolic reactions
(b) Anabolic reactions
(c) Amphibolic reactions
(d) None of these

187. Entner-Doudoroff pathway is found in

(a) Aerobic prokaryotes
(b) Anaerobic prokaryotes
(c) Both (a) and (b)
(d) Aerobic eukaryotes

188. Anoxygenic photosynthetic bacteria oxidize

(a) Water
(b) Oxgyen
(c) Sulfide
(d) Ammonia

189. Which of the following(s) is/are the products of the light reactions of photosynthesis?

(a) ATP only
(b) NADPH only
(c) ATP and O_2 only
(d) ATP, NADPH, and O_2

190. Which of the following catalyze liberation of orthophosphate from organic P compounds and inorganic pyrophosphate ?

(a) Alkaline phosphates (b) Oxidoreductase

(c) Protease (d) Hydrogenase

191. For each glucose molecule broken down, there are _________ number of reduced coenzymes to be oxidized.

(a) 12 (b) 8

(c) 6 (d) 4

192. As the electron flow through the chains, much of their free energy is conserved in the form of ATP. This process is called

(a) Oxidative phosphorylation (b) Electromotive potential

(c) Dehydrogenations (d) None of these

193. Digestive reactions where large molecules are broken down into smaller ones are referred as

(a) Anabolism (b) Catabolism

(c) Metabolism (d) Biosynthesis

194. Phosphate regulation has been observed in the production of

(a) Alkaloids (b) Antibiotics

(c) Gibberelins (d) All of these

195. Most of the energy in aerobic respiration of glucose is captured by

(a) Substrate-level phosphorylation

(b) Electron transport of electrons from NADH

(c) Long-chain fatty acid oxidation

(d) The enzyme formic-hydrogen lyase

196. During the reduction phase of the Calvin cycle, phosphoglyceric acid is reduced to _________ utilizing _________ as the reduction source.

(a) Phosphoglyceraldehyde; $NADPH^{+}H^{+}$

(b) Phosphoglyceraldehyde; $NADH^{+}H^{+}$

(c) Ribulose 1,5 - bisphosphate; $NADH^{+}H^{+}$

(d) Pyruvic acid; $NADPH^{+}H^{+}$

197. In order to get inorganic phosphorus into organic compounds, the phosphate ion is incorporated via

(a) Substrate level phosphorylation (b) Oxidative phosphorylation

(c) Both (a) and (b) (d) DNA

198. The phosphate inhibition in the clavine formation with *Claviceps* SD58, can be counteracted by the addition of

(a) Alanine (b) Methionine
(c) Tryptophan (d) Lysine

199. The major route for incorporation of ammonia (NH_4^+) into organic compounds is via

(a) Reduction of pyruvate or alpha-ketoglutarate by enzymes
(b) Atmospheric nitrogen fixation
(c) Oxidation of pyruvate
(d) All of these

200. The specific enzyme/(s) of the glyoxylate cycle is/are

(a) Isocitrate lyase (b) Malate synthase
(c) Both (a) and (b) (d) Anaplerotic

201. If ΔG of a chemical reaction has a negative value, the reaction

(a) Releases energy (b) Requires energy
(c) Both (a) and (b) (d) None of these

202. The catabolic reaction, pentose-phosphate exists in

(a) Prokaryotic cells (b) Eukaryotic cells
(c) Prokaryotic and eukaryotic cells both (d) None of these

203. Entner - Doudoroff pathway is not found in

(a) Aerobic prokaryotes (b) Anaerobic prokaryotes
(c) Both (a) and (b) (d) Eukaryotes

204. Aerobic catabolism of glucose yields how much energy (ATP synthesized) relative to glucose fermentation?

(a) Slightly less (b) About the same
(c) Twice as much (d) More than 10 times as much

205. The bacteriochlorophylls used by the anoxygenic bacteria have absorbance maxima located in the __________ portion(s) of the spectrum.

(a) Green (b) Blue
(c) Ultraviolet (d) Infrared

206. The relationship between an oxidation-reduction potential difference and the standard free energy change is (where n is the number of moles of electron transferred, F= Faraday's constant and E°= standard oxidation-reduction potential difference)

(a) $\Delta G° = -nFE°$ (b) $\Delta G° = nFE°$
(c) $\Delta G° = -nF\ln E°$ (d) $\Delta G° = nF\ln E°$

207. ATPase

(a) Synthesizes ATP, coupled to transfer of extracellular protons into the cell

(b) Extrudes protons from the cell coupled to the hydrolysis of ATP to ADP

(c) Is the enzyme that incorporates ATP into messenger RNA

(d) Carries out each of the reactions indicated in (a) and (b)

208. Which of the following is responsible for phosphate solubilization?

(a) *Streptococcus* (b) *Streptomyces*

(c) *Bacillus* (d) *Clostridium*

209. Phosphate deregulated mutants are

(a) Less sensitive to phosphate regulation

(b) Moderately sensitive to phosphate regulation

(c) Highly sensitive to phosphate regulation

(d) None of these

210. The mechanism of passive or facilitated diffusion require

(a) Metabolic energy

(b) Concentration of solute against an electrochemical gradient

(c) Accumulation of solute against an electrochemical gradient

(d) Accumulation or concentration of solute against an electrochemical gradient

211. Nitrogen fixation is a process that requires

(a) Energy (b) An anaerobic environment

(c) Both (a) and (b) (d) An aerobic environment

212. Bacteriochlorophyll differs from chlorophyll in what way?

(a) The chelated metal in bacteriochlorophyll is not Mg

(b) There are chemical differences between the two chlorophyll in their side (R) groups

(c) They have different absorption spectra

(d) Both (b) and (c)

213. Radioisotopes are frequently used in the study of cells. Assume a culture of E. coli is grown in a culture medium containing radioactive sulphur. At the end of 48 hours, it is expected to find the radioactive label located in

(a) DNA (b) Enzymes

(c) RNA (d) All of these

214. In the time since *E. coli* and *Salmonella* diverged evolutionarily

(a) There has been little change in either genome

(b) *E. coli* has acquired many genes via horizontal transfer

(c) *E. coli* has lost approximately 50 per cent of its genome

(d) None of these

215. Which of the following theory is supported by the genomic sequence of the obligate intracellular parasite *Rickettsia prowazekii* ?

(a) Parasitic bacteria have very large genomes

(b) Parasites have a definite genomic sequence similar to viruses

(c) Mitochondria have evolved from endosymbiotic bacteria

(d) All bacteria evolved from viruses

216. The physical nature of genomes is studied under

(a) Structural genomics (b) Comparative genomics

(c) Proteo genomics (d) Functional genomics

217. The species of bacteria, which possesses 250 genes for lipid biosynthesis is

(a) *M. genitalium* (b) *M. tuberculosis*

(c) *E. coli* (d) *H. influenzae*

218. Why the bacterium *Treponema pallidum* is difficult to culture?

(a) Because it requires a great deal of water to reproduce

(b) Because it is unable to use carbohydrates as an energy source

(c) Because it lacks the genes needed for TCA cycle and oxidative phosphorylation

(d) Because it requires extremely low temperature at which water freezes

219. What is the range of minimum set of genes required for life?

(a) 50-100 genes (b) 250-350 genes

(c) 1000-1500 genes (d) 1500-2000 genes

220. The flow of genetic material in microbial cells usually takes place from

(a) RNA through DNA to proteins

(b) Proteins through RNA to DNA

(c) DNA through RNA to proteins

(d) None of these

221. Which of the following is used for determining the location of specific genes within the genome?

(a) Genomics (b) Annotation

(c) Cloning (d) Proteomics

222. Proteomics is

(a) The study of algal genomes

(b) A branch of quantum physics dealing with proteins

(c) The study of formation of lipo-protein in animals

(d) The study of the entire collection of proteins expressed by an organism

223. Which of the following is concerned with the management and analysis of biological data using computers?

(a) Biophysics
(b) Bioinformatics
(c) Genomics
(d) Biomechanics

224. Which type of genomics studies the transcripts and proteins expressed by a genome?

(a) Comparative genomics
(b) Structural genomics
(c) Proteo genomics
(d) Functional genomics

225. Which of the following is the study of the molecular organization of genomes, their information content and the gene products they encode?

(a) Genetics
(b) Ergonomics
(c) Genomics
(d) Bioinformatics

226. The word, used for the small solid supports onto which are spotted hundreds of thousands of tiny drops of DNA that can be used to screen gene expression, is

(a) Southern blot
(b) Cloning library
(c) DNA microarrays
(d) Northern blot

227. Which of the following organisms has the smallest genome?

(a) *H. influenzae*
(b) *M. genitalium*
(c) *M. tuberculosis*
(d) None of these

228. Studies of similarities and differences among the genomes of multiple organisms is carried out in

(a) Comparative genomics
(b) Proteomics
(c) Functional genomics
(d) Structural genomics

229. Why Deinococcus radiodurans is able to survive massive exposure to radiation?

(a) Because it produces a thick shell which acts as a shield from the radiation

(b) Because it has unique DNA repair mechanisms

(c) Because its cellwall contains radioactive elements

(d) Because it has many copies of genes encoding DNA repair

230. The plasmid-mediated properties is/are

(a) Fermentation of lactose
(b) Production of enterotoxin
(c) Resistance to antibiotics
(d) All of these

231. In the extracellular medium, DNA-degrading enzymes would likely be to prevent transfer of DNA by

(a) Conjugal transfer by a self-transmissible plasmid
(b) Generalized phage transduction
(c) Natural transformation
(d) None of the above

232. What is the term used for a segment of DNA with one or more genes in the centre and the two ends carrying inverted repeat sequences of nucleotides?

(a) Plasmid
(b) Transposon
(c) Insertion sequence
(d) None of these

233. The plasmids can be eliminated from a cell by the process known as

(a) Curing
(b) Breaking
(c) Fixing
(d) Expulsion

234. Recombination of virus genomes occurs

(a) By transduction
(b) By transription
(c) Simultaneous infection of a host cell by two viruses with homologous chromosomes
(d) By transformation

235. The type of recombination that commonly occurs between a pair of homologous DNA sequences is,

(a) Mutagenic recombination
(b) Site-specific recombination
(c) Replicative recombination
(d) General recombination

236. Which of the following statement describes plasmids?

(a) Another name for a protoplast
(b) A complex membrane structure that covers the chromosome of bacteria
(c) Small, circular DNA molecules that can exist independently of chromosomes commonly found in bacteria
(d) None of the above

237. In lysogeny,

(a) A bacteriophage transfers bacterial DNA
(b) Bacteria take up double stranded DNA from the environment

(c) DNA-degrading enzymes in the extracellular medium would stop the process
(d) A bacteriophage genome is integrated into the bacterial genome

238. A microarray differs from a gene fusion in that, it

(a) Carries DNA segments from many different genes
(b) Is not constructed by cloning
(c) Gives direct measurement of mRNA level
(d) All of the above

239. Who discovered transposons (jumping genes)?

(a) Abelson (b) Harvey
(c) McClintock (d) Griffith

240. Which type of plasmid can exist with or without being integrated into the host's chromosome?

(a) Medisome (b) Lisosome
(c) Lysogen (d) Episome

241. The main difference between a self-transmissible and a mobilizable plasmid is that the self-transmissible plasmid

(a) Transfers both strands of the plasmid DNA
(b) Carries genes encoding the mating apparatus
(c) Transfers antibiotic resistance genes
(d) Usually has a transposon inserted into it

242. Which of the following is the cause for drug resistance in tuberculosis?

(a) Mutation (b) Transduction
(c) Transformation (d) Conjugation

243. The transposase gene encodes an enzyme that facilitate

(a) Viral replication within a genome
(b) General recombination
(c) Site-specific integration of transposable elements
(d) None of the above

244. The term used for plasmids possessing both RTF and *r* determinants is

(a) Non self-transmissible plasmids (b) Non conjugative plasmids
(c) Conjugative plasmids (d) None of the above

245. Diagnostic DNA probes have been developed for

(a) *Mycobacterium tuberculosis* (b) Hepatitis B virus
(c) Human immunodeficiency virus (d) All of the above

246. Which of the following statement(s) is/are true in regards to F^+ x F^- mating events?

(a) DNA is transferred from F^- to F^+ cells

(b) DNA is transferred from F^+ to F^- cells

(c) No DNA is transferred because F^- cells are unable to perform conjugation

(d) No DNA is transferred because F^+ cells are unable to perform conjugation

247. Which of the following type of recombination does not require homologous sequences and is important for the integration of viral genomes into bacterial chromosomes?

(a) Mutagenic recombimation
(b) Site-specific recombination
(c) Replicative recombination
(d) General recombination

248. What information can be generated by interrupted mating experiments?

(a) Levels of DNA homology
(b) Bacterial genome maps
(c) DNA nucleotide sequences
(d) Proteomics of the bacteria

249. Which of the following transport bacterial DNA to other bacteria via bacteriophages?

(a) Conjugation
(b) Transduction
(c) Transformation
(d) Translation

250. When composite transposons are formed

(a) A small deletion occurs in the transposase gene of an IS element

(b) A small deletion occurs in the transposase gene of an IS element and plasmid is integrated

(c) An IS element integrates with another IS element with the help of a plasmid

(d) Two IS elements integrate into a chromosome with only a small distance separating them

251. Which of the following plamids do not possess information for self transfer to another cell?

(a) Cryptic plasmids
(b) Conjugative plasmids
(c) Non-conjugative plasmids
(d) None of these

252. The term used for acquisition of naked DNA from its environment and its incorporation in their genome by a bacterium is

(a) Transformation
(b) Lysogenic conversion
(c) Conjugation
(d) Transduction

253. What is term used for a bacterial cell that is able to take up naked DNA?

(a) Complementary
(b) Liable
(c) Competent
(d) Infected

254. Penicillin resistance in *staphylococci* is acquired due to

(a) Conjugation (b) Mutation
(c) Transformation (d) Transduction

255. The plasmid which makes the host more pathogenic is

(a) F factors (b) Metabolic plasmid
(c) Virulence plasmid (d) None of these

256. The expression of gene X (which has promoter Px) is to be monitored. A gene fusion construction for carrying this work will

(a) Have Px but not the rest of the X coding region
(b) Have the promoter of *lacZ* or some other reporter gene
(c) Allow to monitor the expression of all genes with a promoter similar in sequence to Px
(d) Give the same information as from a microarray

257. The transducing particles carry only specific portions of the bacterial genome in which of the following transduction?

(a) Specialized transduction (b) General transduction
(c) Abortive transduction (d) None of these

258. The correct term for the transfer of genetic material between bacteria in direct physical contact is

(a) Conjugation (b) Transformation
(c) Replication (d) Transduction

259. Plasmid that carries genes encoding enzymes, which degrade substances such as aromatic compounds, pesticides or sugar are

(a) F factors (b) Metabolic plasmid
(c) Virulence plasmid (d) None of these

260. R factors involved in plant-microbe interactions are

(a) Plant proteins (b) Bacterial proteins
(c) Essential for transfer of DNA to plant cells (d) Also called opines

261. Which of the following is used by microbial genetisists as a tool?

(a) Bacteriophage (b) Plasmids
(c) Transposable elements (d) All of these

262. Which of the following type of recombination does not require homologous sequences and is utilized by mobile genetic elements that move about chromosomes?

(a) Mutagenic recombimation (b) Site-specific recombination
(c) Replicative recombination (d) General recombination

263. Which of the following term describes the relationship between a virus and host where no new viral particles are produced and the viral genome is replicated along with host chromosome?

(a) Lysogeny (b) Lysis
(c) Transformation (d) Conjugation

264. Inverted repeat sequences at each end and a gene encoding transposase is contained in which of the following transposable element?

(a) Composite transposon (b) Insertion element
(c) Virus (d) Plasmid

265. F factor plasmids play a major role in

(a) Conjugation (b) Replication
(c) Transduction (d) Trasnscription

266. Which of the following genetic elements carry the genes required for integration into host chromosomes?

(a) Replicon (b) Plasmids
(c) Transposons (d) Tandons

267. The chromosomal genes, possessing fertility factor is known as

(a) R factor (b) F prime factor
(c) HFr (d) F factor

268. Which of the following statement can describe horizontal transfer?

(a) The synthesis of protein in RNA
(b) The transmission of genetic information from one independent, mature organism to another
(c) The transmission of genetic information from parent to offspring
(d) The synthesis of RNA from a DNA template

269. Which of the following characteristic of the Rotavirus was important for the construction of the Rotashield vaccine?

(a) The possession of a segmented RNA genome
(b) A limited number of capsule types
(c) The ability of monkey Rotavirus strains to cause serious illness (diarrhea) in human beings
(d) The ability of the Rotavirus to be transmitted faster

270. Plastic implants can pose a serious nosocomial infection problem because

(a) Phagocytes have trouble moving on the plastic surface

(b) Phagocytes have trouble engulfing bacteria embedded in a biofilm

(c) Infected implants usually have to be surgically removed

(d) All of the above

Answers

1	(a)	21	(a)	41	(a)	61	(d)
2	(b)	22	(a)	42	(b)	62	(c)
3	(d)	23	(d)	43	(d)	63	(c)
4	(c)	24	(c)	44	(d)	64	(a)
5	(d)	25	(b)	45	(d)	65	(c)
6	(a)	26	(d)	46	(c)	66	(d)
7	(b)	27	(b)	47	(c)	67	(b)
8	(c)	28	(b)	48	(a)	68	(a)
9	(c)	29	(d)	49	(a)	69	(b)
10	(c)	30	(d)	50	(c)	70	(a)
11	(c)	31	(d)	51	(c)	71	(d)
12	(c)	32	(a)	52	(d)	72	(b)
13	(b)	33	(a)	53	(c)	73	(d)
14	(c)	34	(c)	54	(c)	74	(c)
15	(c)	35	(a)	55	(d)	75	(c)
16	(c)	36	(d)	56	(d)	76	(d)
17	(b)	37	(a)	57	(a)	77	(d)
18	(c)	38	(a)	58	(c)	78	(a)
19	(a)	39	(b)	59	(c)	79	(c)
20	(d)	40	(a)	60	(a)	80	(d)
81	(d)	115	(b)	149	(c)	183	(a)
82	(c)	116	(b)	150	(a)	184	(a)
83	(b)	117	(b)	151	(d)	185	(c)
84	(d)	118	(d)	152	(b)	186	(c)
85	(d)	119	(c)	153	(c)	187	(c)
86	(c)	120	(c)	154	(d)	188	(c)

87	(a)	121	(b)	155	(a)	189	(d)
88	(d)	122	(a)	156	(b)	190	(a)
89	(b)	123	(d)	157	(a)	191	(a)
90	(c)	124	(b)	158	(d)	192	(a)
91	(a)	125	(b)	159	(a)	193	(b)
92	(c)	126	(a)	160	(c)	194	(d)
93	(b)	127	(c)	161	(a)	195	(b)
94	(c)	128	(b)	162	(a)	196	(a)
95	(c)	129	(b)	163	(d)	197	(c)
96	(c)	130	(d)	164	(b)	198	(c)
97	(b)	131	(a)	165	(c)	199	(a)
98	(a)	132	(d)	166	(a)	200	(c)
99	(a)	133	(b)	167	(a)	201	(a)
100	(b)	134	(b)	168	(a)	202	(c)
101	(d)	135	(c)	169	(b)	203	(d)
102	(d)	136	(a)	170	(b)	204	(d)
103	(d)	137	(b)	171	(a)	205	(d)
104	(c)	138	(b)	172	(b)	206	(a)
105	(a)	139	(a)	173	(a)	207	(d)
106	(d)	140	(d)	174	(a)	208	(c)
107	(d)	141	(c)	175	(a)	209	(a)
108	(d)	142	(c)	176	(c)	210	(a)
109	(c)	143	(b)	177	(b)	211	(c)
110	(b)	144	(a)	178	(c)	212	(d)
111	(d)	145	(c)	179	(b)	213	(b)
112	(a)	146	(a)	180	(c)	214	(c)
113	(b)	147	(d)	181	(a)	215	(c)
114	(c)	148	(d)	182	(a)	216	(a)

217	(b)	231	(c)	245	(d)	259	(b)
218	(c)	232	(b)	246	(b)	260	(a)
219	(b)	233	(a)	247	(b)	261	(d)
220	(c)	234	(c)	248	(b)	262	(c)
221	(b)	235	(d)	249	(b)	263	(a)

222	(d)	236	(c)	250	(d)	264	(b)
223	(b)	237	(d)	251	(c)	265	(a)
224	(d)	238	(d)	252	(a)	266	(c)
225	(c)	239	(c)	253	(c)	267	(b)
226	(c)	240	(d)	254	(d)	268	(b)
227	(b)	241	(b)	255	(c)	269	(a)
228	(a)	242	(a)	256	(a)	270	(d)
229	(d)	243	(c)	257	(a)		
230	(d)	244	(c)	258	(a)		

Chapter 39
Gene Expression

1. **One gene one enzyme theory was proposed by**
   (a) Temin and Baltimore (b) Watson and Crick
   (c) Robert and Koch (d) Beadle and Tatum
2. **Formation of RNA from DNA is known as**
   (a) Transcription (b) Translation
   (c) Replication (d) Recombination
3. **Mendelian recombination are due to**
   (a) Linkage
   (b) Independent assortment of genes
   (c) Mutation
   (d) Dominant characters
4. **Unwinding of DNA is done by**
   (a) Topoisomerase (b) Exonuclease
   (c) Helicase (d) Ligase
5. **Fluid mosaic model of cell membrane was given by**
   (a) Beadle and Tatum (b) Singer and Nicolson
   (c) Watson and Crick (d) Robertson and Miller
6. **The name of Temin and Baltimore is associated with**
   (a) Photorespiration (b) RNA
   (c) Reverse transcription (d) All of these
7. **Genes are responsible for the growth and differentiation in an organism through regulation**
   (a) Of translocation (b) Of transformation
   (c) Of translation and transcription (d) Transduction

8. **Normally DNA molecule has A-T, G-C paring however these bases can exist in alternative valeancy status, occurring to rearrangement called**
   (a) Point mutation (b) Analog substitution
   (c) From shift mutation (d) Tautomerisational mutation

9. **The cells which help in folding or rolling or leaves in grasses, are called**
   (a) Trichoplast (b) Guard cells
   (c) Bulliform cells (d) Mucilagenaus cells

10. **Cell wall of gram positive bacteria is made up of**
   (a) Murein (b) Cellulose
   (c) Lepid and protein (d) Cellulose and lipid

11. **The no of hydrogen bonds b/w adenine and thymine in DNA molecule are**
   (a) Two (b) Three
   (c) Four (d) Eight

12. **Plasmid are**
   (a) Nucleoid
   (b) New types of micro-organism
   (c) Bi-linear chromosome
   (d) Extra chromosomal circular material

13. **In which of the following stages the chromosomes appear thin long and thread like**
   (a) Zygotene (b) Pachytene
   (c) Leptotene (d) Diakenensis

14. **Longitudinal quality of each chromosome of homologous pair become clearly evident showing formation of four chromatids from each bivalent at:**
   (a) Diplotene (b) Zygotene
   (c) Pachytene (d) Diakinensis

15. **A cell become turgid when placed in**
   (a) Isotonic solution (b) Sypertonic solution
   (c) Hypotonic solution (d) None of these

16. **Synapsis is the characteristic of:**
   (a) Leptotene (b) Zygotene
   (c) Pachytene (d) Diplotene

17. **Which of these ion is involved in the closing and opening of stomata?**
   (a) Mg^{2+} (b) Na^{2+}
   (c) Fe^{2+} (d) K^{+}

18. As a tree grows older, which of the following increase more rapidly in thickness?

(a) Phloem (b) Cortex

(c) Heart wood (d) Sap Wood

19. For determining the c-terminal amino acid of polypephde chain the reagent that would be useful is:

(a) Trypsis (b) Carboxypeptidase

(c) Phenyl isothiocyanate (d) 1 (N) HCl

20. Which statement is incorrect?

(a) Solubility of polypeptide depends upon relative polarity of their R group

(b) Higher ionizable group in polypeptides make it more soluble

(c) Isoelectric point of histones is very high (about 10.8)

(d) Selenocysteine is derived from cysteine

21. Molecular weight of an unknown protein can be found out by

(a) Electrophoresis

(b) Ion-exchange chromatography

(c) Affinity chromatography

(d) None of the above technique

22. N-terminal amino acids are usually determined by sanger's method using

(a) Ninhydrin reagent

(b) Fluro-2,4 dinitrobenzene/ dansylchloride

(c) Hydrazene

(d) Concentrated nitric acid

23. A mixture of lysine, aspartic acid tyrosine and alanine is passed through an anion exchange coloumn at pH 8.0. what is the likely order of elution and amino acids when eluted with a buffer of reducing pH gradient?

(a) Tyr, Lys, Asp, Ala (b) Lys, Ala, Asp, Tyr

(c) Asp, Tyr, Ala, Lys (d) Lys, Tyr, Ala, Asp

24. The closest estimate for the number of amino acid residues in a protein with a molecular weight of 85 KDa is

(a) 710 (b) 7100

(c) 8500 (d) 85

25. Which one of the following bonds in proteins has a partial double bond character?

(a) Cα-c (b) Cα-N

(c) C-N (d) C-O

26. Cleavage of the following peptide with chymotrypsin +H_3-Gly-Arg-Ala-Ser-Phe- Gly-Asn-Lys-Try-Glu-Val-COO^- results in

(a) 2 fragments (b) 3 fagments
(c) 4 fragments (d) None of above

27. The average molecular weight of an amino acid in a protein is

(a) 125 (b) 120
(c) 110 (d) 137

28. Which of the following peptides can be easily detected by absorbance at 280 nm?

1. Leu-Tyr-Met-Ala-Glu **2. Ser-Thr-Trp-Val-Ile-Leu**
3. Ac-Ala-Glu-Gin-Ser-Asp-Lys **4. Thr-Tyr-Trp-Val-Ile**

(a) 1, 2 and 4 (b) 1 and 4
(c) 2 and 3 (d) 2 and 4

29. Two dimensional (2-(d) gel electrophoresis performed under denaturing conditions can be used to separate protein according to which of the following characteristics?

	First Dimension	*Second Dimension*
(a)	Sub unit Mol. weight	Density
(b)	Density	Charge
(c)	Amino acid composition	Charge
(d)	Isoelectric point	Sub unit mo. weight

30. The catabolism of haemoglobin

(a) Involves the removal of the phytol chain
(b) Involves the oxidative cleavage of the porphyrin ring
(c) Results in the liberation of CO_2
(d) None of the above

31. Disulphide bonds most often stabilize the native structure of

(a) Extra cellular protein (b) Dimeric proteins
(c) Intracelular proteins (d) Multisubunit proteins

32. The helices in the amino acid super secondary structure are held together primary by

(a) Charge-charge tinteraction
(b) Covalent cross links
(c) Favorable R group interactions
(d) Main chain hydrogen bonding

33. The mirror image of right handed α-helix with all L-amino acids well appear as

(a) Left handed α-helix with L-amino acid

(b) Left handed α-helix with D-amino acid

(c) Ritht handed α-helix with D-amino acid

(d) Right handed α-helix with D-amino acid

34. The peptide bond in proteins is

(a) Planar, but rotates to three preferred dihedral angles

(b) Non-polar, but rotates to three preferred, dihedral angels

(c) Non-polar and fixed in a trans conformation

(d) Planar and usually found in a transformations

35. A competitive inhibitor

(a) Increase the km of an enzyme

(b) Decreases the km of an enzyme

(c) Increases both vimax and the km of an enzyme

(d) None of above

36. Characteristic unique of DNA is

(a) Denaturation and renaturation

(b) Polymer complex

(c) Replication

(d) Resistance to temperature charge

37. A solution contain DNA polymerase I, Mg^{2+} salts of dATP, dGTP, dCTP and dTTP and an appropriate buffer which of the following DNA molecule would serve as a temperate for DNA synthesis when added to this solution

(a) A single stranded closed circles

(b) A single stranded closed circle base paired to a shorter linear strand with 3-terminal hydroxyl

(c) A single stranded closed circle base paired to a shorter linear strand with 3′ terminal phosphate

(d) A double standard closed circle

38. Approximately how many O kazaki fragments are synthesized during one round of replication of the E. cole geneme

(a) 5000 to 10000 (b) 4×10^6

(c) 2500 to 5000 (d) 2

39. In prokaryotes the lagging primers are removed by

(a) 3′ to 5′ exonuclease (b) DNA lo gase

(c) DNA polymerase I (d) DNA polymerase II

40. The essential initiator protein at the *E. coli* origin of replication is

(a) Dna A (b) Dna B

(c) Dna C (d) Dna E

41. Synthesis of peptide bond is catalyzed by

(a) A site of ribosome (b) P site of ribosome

(c) 23s rRNA (d) TRNA

42. Which of the following is not an antibacterial antibiotic?

(a) Tetracycline (b) Streptomycin

(c) Nystatin (d) Nali dixic acid

43. Which site of ribosome first fill up by tRNA carrying initiating amino acid?

(a) Peptidyl site (b) Amino acetyl site

(c) Either P site or A site (d) None of these

44. Which of the following group of amino acids have maximum codons?

(a) Methionine, tryptophan

(b) Leusene, serine, valene

(c) Leusine, serine, argenine

(d) Tryptophan, methionine arginine

45. What is ubiquitin?

P) A subvnit of the electron transport chain coenzyme Q ubiquinone.

Q) A generic name for the most abundant protein in chloroplast, rubisco

R) A polypeptide involved in making protein for degradation

S) A polypeptide that modifies a fraction of H2A histone molecule during the cell

(a) P, Q (b) Q, R

(c) R, S (d) P, Q, R, S

46. Chloramphenicol inhibited

(a) Cell wall synthesis in baiteria

(b) Protein synthesis on 70s ribosome

(c) Protein synthesis on 80s ribosome

(d) DNA replication

47. How many polypeptide chain can be formed simultaneously by a given ribosome

(a) One

(b) Up to 30

(c) Variable, depending on the length of the *m*RNA

(d) Variable, depending both on length or *m*RNA temperature

48. Three of the four eukaryotic rRNAs are synthesized from a single transcription unit consisting of the rDNA. Which one of the following does not belong to this group.

(a) 58s (b) 5s

(c) 18s (d) 28s

49. Shine dalgarno sequence of mRNA is helpful (n)

(a) Recognition of 50s ribosomal subunit

(b) Recognition of 60s ribosomal unit

(c) Recognition of 50s rRNA

(d) Recognition of 30s subunit of ribosome

50. Noncoding DNA is eukanyotic cell do not enclude

(a) Introns (b) Pseudogenes

(c) Simplc sequence DNA (d) Mobile genetic elements

51. Arginine and lysine are found in what form

(a) Negative ion (b) Positive ion

(c) Negative ion (d) Positive ion

52. Which of the following cell unable to undergo mitosis on which

(a) Containing polytene chromosome

(b) Contain lambrush chromosome

(c) Containing B-chromosome

(d) All of these

53. Nucleolus is chemically composed of

(a) RNA, DNA and protein

(b) RNA and protein only

(c) DNA and protein only

(d) Nucleic acid, protein and phospholipid

54. Chromosomal puffs (Balbiani rings) are active site of

(a) RNA synthesis (b) DNA replication

(c) Lipid synthesis (d) Polysachandi synthesis

55. Telomeres are present in eukaryotic genomes at the chromosomal ends.

(a) As selfish DNA

(b) To protect from breakdown

(c) To encode essential genes envolved in ageing

(d) To silence genes at the ends of chromosomes

56. Which of the following are genes found in all retro viruses?

P) Gag Q) Pol R) Env S) onc

(a) P, Q

(b) P,S

(c) R,S

(d) P,Q,R

57. All histones undergo post-translational modification of specific amino acids. These modification

P) Alter the change of the histone moleculs

Q) One permanent

R) Occur (in part) on the N-terminal arms of the histones, which are though to extend out from the core

S) Occur at specific time during the cell cycle

(a) P,Q

(b) P,S

(c) P,R,S

(d) P,Q,S

58. Which of the following mRNA lack poly A tail.

(a) Ferritin

(b) Interferon

(c) Insulin

(d) None of above

59. DNA can act as a messenger at the ribosome only

(a) In prions

(b) In vitro

(c) With reverse transcription

(d) Never

60. In eukaryotic the enzyme that primarily transcribes the nucleolar organizer is

(a) RNA polymerase I

(b) RNA polymerase II

(c) Primase

(d) Reverse transcriptase

61. Polymerase chain reaction (PCR) is used to

(a) Amplify or make more copies of a small amount of DNA

(b) Cleave bacterial plasmid

(c) Seal sticky ends

(d) Identify target plasmid

62. Which is the correct order for 3 steps of polymerase chain reaction (PCR)

(a) Denaturation of DNA, annealing of primers, primer extension

(b) Primer extension, annealing of primer, denaturation of DNA

(c) Annealing of primer, primer extension, denaturation of DNA

(d) All of these

63. In each cycle of PCR the quantity of the DNA is

(a) Tripled
(b) Doubled
(c) Quarter
(d) Increased by 50 per cent

64. What is the purpose of the southern blot?

(a) Amplify DNA

(b) Identify a specific gene in a DNA sequence

(c) Seal the sticky ends of DNA cut with restriction enzyme

(d) Separate DNA fragments upon change

65. In preliminary screening of a clone library, it common to use

(a) Restriction enzyme
(b) Dyes
(c) Antibiotics
(d) Radiaction

66. Plasmids usually contain genes for antibiotics resistance which statement is true in regards to screening a clone library?

(a) All bacterial colonies that contain plasmids will did in the presence of antibiotics

(b) All bacterial colonies that do not contains plasmids will die in the presence of antibiotics

(c) Only plasmids without genes for antibiotic resistance contain genes of interest

(d) All the above

67. Bacteria protect themselves from viruses by fragmenting viral DNA with

(a) Restriction ligases
(b) Restriction enzyme
(c) Restriction methylase
(d) Vectors

68. In PCR, how are the DNA segments sorted?

(a) Gel electrophoresis
(b) Centrifugation
(c) Chromatography
(d) All of the above

69. When sticky ends are paired, they can be joined by

(a) Restriction enzymes
(b) RNA polymerase
(c) Methylate
(d) DNA ligase

70. Gel electrophoresis separate molecules based upon

(a) Size (b) Shape

(c) Charge (d) All of the above

71. Genetically identical organisms derived from a single genetic source are called

(a) Population (b) Varieties

(c) Sibling species (d) Clones

72. When tryptophan is present in the environment of E. coli the tryptophan binds to the

(a) Trp operon (b) Trp expression

(c) Trp repressor (d) Trp operator

73. Which statement(s) is /are true if tryptophan is present in the environment of E. coli

(a) The repressor is not bound to the operator

(b) RNA polymerase binds to the promoter

(c) Transcription occurs to the operator

(d) The repressor is bound to the operator

74. From time a nucleotide is added as the transcription bubble passes down the DNA, the RNA-DNA complex

(a) Elongates (b) Rotates

(c) Shrinks (d) Disassembles

75. Eukryotic mRNA transcripts are protected from modification by

(a) 5′ caps (b) 5′ poly A tail

(c) 5′ caps (d) 5′-3′ poly tails

76. The order in which nucleotides are moved along the ribosomes binding sites is

(a) APE (b) PEA

(c) EPA (d) EAP

77. In eukaryotes, the start codon also specifies the amino acids

(a) Phenylalanine (b) Valene

(c) Aspartate (d) Methionine

78. The function of RNA is to

(a) Provide a site for polypeptide synthesis

(b) Transport amino acids to the ribosomes

(c) Travel to the ribosome to direct the assembly of polypeptide

(d) Transcribe DNA

79. Enzymes called amino cycle tRNA synthetizes
   (a) Synthesis tRNA
   (b) Attaches amino acids to tRNA
   (c) Strips tRNA from its amino acid in the process of translation
   (d) Destroye excess tRNA molecules

80. In mRNA the "start" sequence is
   (a) UAA (b) UAG
   (c) UGA (d) AUG

81. In mRNA the series of nucleotides ccc specifics
   (a) Serene (b) Prolene
   (c) Alanine (d) Arginine

82. What is the usual sequence of pribnow box?
   (a) TTGACA (b) TATAAT
   (c) UUUUU (d) All the above

83. Following binding to a promoter, RNA polymerase next
   (a) Unwinds a short segment of DNA (b) Nicks one strand of DNA
   (c) Begins to replicate DNA (d) All of these

84. Which of the following components in found is all prokaryotic transcription terminator?
   (a) Rho factor (b) A poly u region
   (c) A hair pin structure (d) All the above

85. Post transcriptional modification of RNA is more common in
   (a) Prokaryotes (b) Eukaryotes
   (c) All of the above (d) None of these

86. Which structure is found an eukaryotic mRNA but not prokaryotic mRNA
   (a) 3′ poly a Tail (b) 5′ cap
   (c) All of the above (d) None of these

87. Which regions of enterrupted gene code for RNA that will be present in the final RNA product
   (a) Intron (b) Exons
   (c) Promoter (d) All of these

88. **What is a ribozyme?**
   (a) A protein that synthesizes RNA
   (b) An RNA molecule that catalyzes a self splicing reaction
   (c) A DNA molecule that acts as a template for RNA synthesis
   (d) All of the above

89. **What is happen during amino acid activation**
   (a) A methyl group is attached to an amino acid
   (b) An amino acid is bound to mRNA
   (c) An amino acid is bound to tRNA
   (d) All of the above

90. **Which protein of tRNA molecule is complementary to the mRNA triplet encoding a particular amino acid?**
   (a) D arm
   (b) Anticodon triplet
   (c) Amino acid stem
   (d) All of the above

91. **Most prokaryotic proteins begin with this modified amino acid**
   (a) N-formylleucene
   (b) N-formyl methionine
   (c) N-formylserine
   (d) All of above

92. **The most common initiator codon is**
   (a) GUA
   (b) UAA
   (c) AUG
   (d) All the above

93. **Which part of translation envolves the addition of amino acids to an existing polypephade chain?**
   (a) Initiation
   (b) Elongation
   (c) Termination
   (d) All the above

94. **What molecule catalyzes the transpeptidation reaction?**
   (a) Pepatidyl transferase
   (b) RNA polymerase
   (c) DNA ligase
   (d) All the above

95. **Aminoacyle tRNA binds to which site of the ribosome during elongation**
   (a) P-site
   (b) A site
   (c) E site
   (d) All the above

96. **Which of the following is not a nonsense codon**
   (a) AGU
   (b) UAA
   (c) UGA
   (d) All the above

97. What is the role of molecular chaperones?

(a) To facilitate binding of ribosomes to mRNA

(b) To degrade newly synthesized polypeptides that contain inaccurate sequence

(c) To aid a newly synthesized polypeptide in folding to its proper shape

(d) All the above

98. An enzyme whose amount is reduced by the presence of an end product are:

(a) Inducible enzymes (b) Repressible enzymes

(c) Corepressors (d) All the above

99. A small molecule that causes the increases in levels of an inducible enzyme

(a) Repressor (b) Corepressor

(c) Inducer (d) All the above

100. Which is the most specific recombinant DNA library?

(a) Genomic (b) Protein

(c) CDNA (d) Chromosomal

101. Which of the following vectors can carry the largest insect?

(a) Phages (b) Macro plasmeds

(c) Plasmeds (d) YAC and BACS

102. The types of vectors based on the fertility plasmid (F factor) are:

(a) Ti plasmeds

(b) Bacterial artificial chromosomes (BACSs)

(c) Yeast and artificial chromosomes

(d) Cosmids

103. Which of the following is an application of PCR technology?

(a) Forensics (b) In vitro mutagenesis

(c) Gene mapping (d) All the above

104. Which of the following is not required for a PCR reaction?

(a) RNA transcriptase (b) A target sequence

(c) Taq polymerase (d) DNTPs

105. cDNA can be synthesized from mRNA by using the following enzyme?

(a) Si nuclease (b) Reverse criptase

(c) DNA polymerase (d) Lysozyme

106. Which type of library would you screen in order to identify the promoter of the hemoglobin gene?

(a) Expression library
(b) Genomic library
(c) CDNA library
(d) None of the above

107. The DNA sequence obtained by both the manual and automatic sequencing corresponds to:

(a) To messenger RNA
(b) The complementary DNA strand
(c) The template DNA strand
(d) The restriction sequence for certain restriction enzymes

108. What sequence on the template strand of DNA corresponds to the first amino acid inserted into a protein?

(a) AUG
(b) ATG
(c) UAC
(d) TAC

109. During translation codon are read from

(a) DNA
(b) *m*RNA
(c) TRNA
(d) RRNA

110. Transcription and translation of a gene composed of 30 nucleotides would from a protein containing no more than how many amino acids?

(a) 10
(b) 15
(c) 30
(d) 60

111. The enzyme peptidyl transferase

(a) Charges *t*RNA
(b) Synthesizes long, artificial *m*RNA
(c) Recognizes the prokaryotic ribosome
(d) Creates peptide bonds b/w amino acid

112. Which of the do not need a primes in order to function

(a) DNA pol I
(b) DNA pol II
(c) DNA pol III
(d) RNA polymerase

113. How many hydrogen bonds from b/w U&A in a Watson-crick pair interaction?

(a) 0
(b) 1
(c) 2
(d) 3

114. End to end joining of DNA

(a) DNA pol I
(b) DNA ligase
(c) DNA pol III
(d) RNA polymerase

115. Only methylated base in mammal is

(a) 7-methyl guanine
(b) Thymine
(c) Methyl adenine
(d) 5 methy cytosine

116. The only nucleoside with base to sugar C-C linkage is

(a) Thymidine
(b) Pseudouridine
(c) Cytidine
(d) Adenosin

117. Repressor molecule bind to the

(a) Promoter
(b) Enhancer
(c) Operator
(d) Hormone response element

118. Which of the following enzyme(s) can remove or insert super coil twist into circular DNA?

(a) Topoisomerases
(b) DNA pol II
(c) Spliceosomes
(d) Helicase

119. Nucleosome

(a) Bind to RNA Pol II
(b) Package prokaryotic DNA
(c) Any only present in prokaryotes
(d) Are composed on an octamer of histone 150 bfg DNA

120. Which of the following mRNAs lack poly a tail?

(a) Ferritin
(b) Interferon
(c) Insulin
(d) None of the above

121. RNA primer is removed from okajaki fragment by

(a) DNA pol I
(b) DNA pol II
(c) DNA pol III
(d) RNA polymerase

122. Histones have an abundance of which of the following amino acid.

(a) Lysine and arginine
(b) Alanine and glutamine
(c) Glycine and glutamine
(d) Arginine and glutamine

123. Which of the following is not cloning vector

(a) Hellicase
(b) PBR 322
(c) SV 40
(d) *E-coli* genomic DNA

Answers

1	(d)	22	(b)	43	(a)	64	(b)
2	(a)	23	(d)	44	(c)	65	(d)
3	(b)	24	(a)	45	(c)	66	(c)
4	(c)	25	(b)	46	(b)	67	(b)
5	(b)	26	(b)	47	(a)	68	(b)
6	(c)	27	(c)	48	(b)	69	(d)
7	(d)	28	(a)	49	(d)	70	(a)
8	(d)	29	(d)	50	(d)	71	(d)
9	(c)	30	(b)	51	(d)	72	(c)
10	(a)	31	(a)	52	(a)	73	(d)
11	(a)	32	(c)	53	(a)	74	(b)
12	(d)	33	(b)	54	(a)	75	(a)
13	(c)	34	(d)	55	(b)	76	(a)
14	(d)	35	(a)	56	(d)	77	(d)
15	(c)	36	(c)	57	(c)	78	(b)
16	(b)	37	(b)	58	(b)	79	(b)
17	(d)	38	(c)	59	(d)	80	(d)
18	(c)	39	(c)	60	(a)	81	(b)
19	(b)	40	(a)	61	(a)	82	(b)
20	(d)	41	(c)	62	(a)	83	(a)
21	(a)	42	(c)	63	(a)	84	(c)

85	**(b)**	**95**	**(b)**	**105**	**(b)**	**115**	**(b)**
86	**(b)**	**96**	**(a)**	**106**	**(b)**	**116**	**(b)**
87	**(b)**	**97**	**(c)**	**107**	**(b)**	**117**	**(c)**
88	**(b)**	**98**	**(b)**	**108**	**(d)**	**118**	**(a)**
89	**(c)**	**99**	**(c)**	**109**	**(b)**	**119**	**(d)**
90	**(b)**	**100**	**(c)**	**110**	**(a)**	**120**	**(b)**
91	**(b)**	**101**	**(d)**	**111**	**(d)**	**121**	**(a)**
92	**(c)**	**102**	**(b)**	**112**	**(d)**	**122**	**(a)**
93	**(a)**	**103**	**(d)**	**113**	**(c)**	**123**	**(a)**
94	**(a)**	**104**	**(a)**	**114**	**(b)**		

www.ingramcontent.com/pod-product-compliance
Ingram Content Group UK Ltd.
Pitfield, Milton Keynes, MK11 3LW, UK
UKHW021450280726
14060UKWH00001BA/337